Dying Well

A guide to enabling a good death

Second edition

Julia Neuberger
Former Chief Executive
King's Fund
London

Radcliffe Publishing
OXFORD • SAN FRANCISCO

Radcliffe Publishing Ltd
18 Marcham Road
Abingdon
Oxon OX14 1AA
United Kingdom

www.radcliffe-oxford.com
Electronic catalogue and worldwide online ordering.

British Library Cataloguing in Publication Data

A catalogue record for this book is available from the British Library.

ISBN 1 85775 940 0

Typeset by Acorn Bookwork Ltd, Salisbury
Printed and bound by TJ International Ltd, Padstow, Cornwall

Contents

Foreword

When Rabbi Julia preached to her South London Liberal congregation about death, they responded, 'Bravo! Now what will you do about it?' Her answer to their challenge was the campaign that built the North London Hospice. The origin, extent and consequences of a taboo about death in the 20th century awaits full assessment, yet Margaret Torrie's Cruse and Dame Cicely Saunders' first hospice began to break it. Since then, the initiatives and team-work of increasing numbers of individuals have started to transform British attitudes to death. Rabbi Julia has not only made the subject of death and dying her own but her leadership in the field of healthcare has helped to ensure the wide salience of the subjects of death and dying.

In giving a warm welcome to the second edition of *Dying Well*, we should recognise how far death has moved up the political agenda in the last five years. The UK government has examined a range of death-related issues including cemeteries, coroners, death registration and certification, retained organs and the Shipman enquiry. This year it will consider advance directives. All these are, in part, responses to newly perceived needs: from within the health services, from the funeral industries, from death- and bereavement-related charities and from reform organisations.

When the sociologist Michael Young turned his spotlight on the role of death in British culture, The Dead Citizens Charter was just part of his overall task, whose scale was assessed by the anthropologist Mary Douglas thus,'He must know that it is difficult to transform a whole culture of embedded reticence. It is hard enough to make a deliberate speech reform; to reform a silence is a tall order.'

Even though we are far better prepared to care for dying and bereaved people than in the 1960s, we need to be, because of the decline of the family and of religion. For generations these two institutions were the drivers of such care. *Dying Well* outlines the next stage, 'What society has to do now is to bring itself to talk more openly about the good death' (p.61). Just over 600 000 people die in the UK each year. If this conversation is to be fruitful, we need far more strategies of collaboration between these families and all the interests providing care.

Dying Well not only encourages this teamwork but argues for death education in our schools, a cause given more prominence this May by the Child Bereavement Trust and others. *Dying Well* welcomes the wider recognition of the spiritual needs of the dying. It also argues for a fuller contribution from the major religions. Rabbi Julia has often noted that the Christian tradition is stronger on care for the sick and dying than for the bereaved. Now she fears that theological discussion of the meaning of death is disappearing from almost all faiths. As Bede's story of King Edwin reminds us, the interpretation of human origin and destiny is a basic contribution of religion to daily life. It should not be discarded.

Attitudes to death are too important for their promotion to be left either to the government or the media. What is required is a wide conversation about the nature, experience and meaning of death at both academic and popular levels. Rabbi Julia's purpose here is to make the dying process life-enhancing for the dying, the bereaved and their carers.

Peter C Jupp
Co-editor of *Mortality*
Visiting Fellow, Department of Sociology
University of Bristol
May 2004

Foreword

Julia Neuberger's book, *Dying Well: A guide to enabling a good death* (2e) is destined to become a classic. It is a rare book that can speak to ordinary members of the public who want to think more about how better to prepare themselves for the death of a loved one, or for their own death. It can serve also as an invaluable guide for healthcare professionals who care for the dying.

What makes this book so remarkable? To begin with, all of us, no matter what our age, gender, class, nationality, religious tradition or none, hope to die well, in reasonable comfort, ripe in years, *compos mentis*, surrounded by our loved ones, at peace with ourselves and the world, feeling we have lived a good life and prepared to return to our ancestors. *Dying Well* (2e) is a well-written book, more of a literary pleasure than a textbook and it affords us a chance to consider our death as a life-enhancing event.

What we yearn for in a book like this is to be in the good company of a deeply intelligent, learned, and compassionate teacher and writer, like Julia Neuberger, who knows a great deal professionally and personally about dying well. It is not incidental to the depth and richness of this book that Julia writes as a mature scholar, a professional Rabbi, the chair of an NHS Trust, and as a daughter – an only child who has had the privilege and responsibility of seeing her mother and father to a good death.

Dying Well (2e) is a humane book, scholarly, intimate, conversant on the issues of the day: the hospice movement, euthanasia, living wills, advance directives and the like; and, at the same time, this is a book written by a professional with a seasoned and generous eye; a woman well acquainted with grief, who captures the details of professional healthcare, grieving and dying, in ways that even the most seasoned of doctors, nurses and other healthcare professionals will find revelatory and informative, and a moving read.

Julia Neuberger knows, for instance, how to approach 'truth-telling' and counseling, how to enable a dying person and their family to be in charge of the most important decisions that they will have to make. Julia states that for many decades healthcare professionals and families have had difficulty talking about dying, grieving, and death. As a consequence, many people feel that they have lost the language with which to speak of death as a meaningful part of life, but the author of *Dying Well* (2e) is not at a loss for words.

Throughout this book, Julia is well spoken, most especially on the subject of religion, a sensitive and important matter intimately related to dying well. Julia is one of the very best in the field, writing on the role of religion in dying well, and *Dying Well* (2e) may well be *the* best book on the subject available to nurses, doctors, and hospice workers; pastoral counselors, Rabbis, priests, and imams; medical students, divinity students and chaplains, all of whom should be required, as a matter of competency, to be religiously informed and religiously literate regarding the role that religion plays (or fails to play) in helping people to die well.

Dying Well (2e) is brilliant for giving us a lively account of the world's religious traditions, according us an excellent grasp of those religious attitudes, rites and rituals that are distinctive to each major tradition. Obviously, not to have this cultural knowledge at hand would leave us woefully unprepared and unskilled to care for people who are dying. Julia Neuberger's voice is rare in that there is nothing parochial in this book, nothing about its presentation of religion that would set the book apart from a general readership, and that is a good thing.

Finally, one cannot fail to be moved by Julia's thoughtful ruminations on funerals, memorial services, and her unparalleled discussion of grief. Reading Julia on the subject of grief, I couldn't put the book down until I had come to its end – she is a powerful writer.

This second edition of *Dying Well* will become an important and major book in the field: its time has come and there is no other book like it, nothing as good. In the courses I teach on death and dying and pastoral care, for divinity students and medical students, *Dying Well* (2e) will become our basic primer. Julia Neuberger has done us a good service and written a wonderful book on dying well, for which we can only be grateful.

Dorothy Austin
Harvard University
Cambridge, Massachusetts
May 2004

Preface

Between the first and second editions of this book, my mother died, my father having died between the first and second drafts of the original edition. Once again, we were blessed with superb care for my mother in her last days, weeks and months, at home, by a dedicated team. More than anything else, more than all the theory, all the observations as a professional rabbi, or chair of an NHS Trust, more than as a theoretician about dying, the experience of the loss of both my parents within a five year period, as an only child where the full responsibility fell on me, has convinced me that we have – at best – a wonderful way of caring for the dying in Britain, if you are lucky enough to live in the right places. And, as I was finishing the work on this second edition, the government announced (26 December 2003) an additional £12 million for training for health professionals in caring for the dying, wherever that might happen, of whatever cause. It is nowhere near enough, but it is a start – the recognition that we cannot all die in hospices, or be cared for by palliative care teams. We do not all die of cancer, MND or AIDS, and our needs, whatever the cause of death, are of paramount importance. Those of us who die of end stage renal failure, or congestive heart disease, are now also, at last, being recognised as deserving high quality care. What we as a family experienced will now, gradually, be rolled out nationwide, if the training and education and encouragement of health professionals is done in the most sympathetic and supportive way as a result of this new initiative.

Meanwhile, I wrote publicly about the deaths of both my parents, partly because neither died of cancer, and partly because I wanted to express my gratitude to the teams, and the system, that ensured both had such good deaths – in their terms, as well as mine, as well as in the terms of the professionals who cared for them. I quote both articles below. When my father died, he had been ill for a long time, and our experience of the care he received from all the professionals involved was extremely positive. Nevertheless, as anyone who has lost a parent, or a spouse, or anyone close to them, will know, it is amazingly painful. One can be left with few regrets and still miss the person terribly, or one can wish one had done more, said more, been there more. Whatever the case, I believe that my work on the two editions of this book, though no other aspect of my life, has been improved by the experience of losing my parents. I hope that it will be helpful both to ordinary members of the public who want to think more about how to prepare themselves for the death of a loved one, or for their own death, and more particularly for healthcare professionals who might find within it some ideas about how death is perceived, and what is felt so strongly, that will help them to care even better for those who are dying under their care. We owe a great debt of gratitude to those who cared for my father and my father-in-law who died 10 weeks after my father, and I append here the article I wrote for the *Health Service Journal* to draw attention to how well we deal with it in this country.

That is important, because I believe there is always room for improvement, but that we have a very high baseline from which to improve our service, and be leaders throughout the world in caring for our dying and those who are left after them.

In the last few months, both my father and my father-in-law have died. It has not been an easy time, but it has been much helped, the whole family has been much helped, by the remarkable support of many staff working within the NHS. I write this as an informed user of services, not from my usual starting point as Chairman of Camden and Islington Community Health Services NHS Trust, though some of the staff who looked after both fathers, and the rest of the family, were from my Trust. I write this because the NHS gets so much flak, and indeed within the NHS as Chairman of a Trust I tend to see so many complaints, that I felt it important to tell the story of what it feels like when things go absolutely right, even though the events concerned, the deaths of much loved fathers, are ones one would wish were not happening.

My father was cared for on and off for the last few years of his life by staff in the cardiology ward of the Royal Free Hospital in Hampstead. He always joked that he had been in every ward of the Free except the maternity wards, but in fact most of his admissions were to the cardiology ward, and they knew him well. When it became clear that there was little more anyone could do for him, the care they gave him was exceptional. Several nurses spent a great deal of time talking to him, asking him how he felt about dying, asking him what his wishes were. When he decided to come home on a Bank Holiday Sunday (why is the NHS so hopeless over Bank Holidays?), when support at home could not be set up, a nurse and a houseman spent hours in the freezing cold, as he sat in my car threatening to drive away, persuading him to stay, until care could be organised. One nurse in parti-

cular befriended him and got his confidence completely, so that he could tell her things he felt he could not tell us.

When he did come home, for what turned out to be the last 28 hours of his life, everyone involved was kind and helpful, from the ambulance men who carried him upstairs and teased him, to the wonderful district nurse who took charge of the situation and helped us organise the next few days, to the Marie Curie nurses who came to be with him constantly, to the GP who helped the district nurse make his bed, and was kindness itself to my mother and me. It was a team effort between professionals and across organisations of a quality I had not witnessed before at such close quarters. It was also an object lesson, as a carer, of how much difference really professional staff, who care passionately about what they do, can make.

My father was a very large man, and it took two or three people to turn him. So we had a visit from the night community nurses, one of whom spent quite some time comforting me. Despite her working in the Trust I chair, I had never met her before. I shall certainly go out with them one night, and watch that remarkable service from a more objective standpoint. For the comfort they brought, late at night when the world is silent, and early in the morning when fears run highest, was considerable.

When it became clear my father was sinking fast, and Alison, the district nurse, and Carol, the Marie Curie nurse, helped me make it clear to my mother – though she did not accept it at the time – the way they did it was a lesson in how to provide care and support well, to my father, my mother, and me. Carol even took my son home at the end of her shift – well beyond the call of any duty.

I wish it were always like this. People might say it was as a result of privilege, because I chair the Trust, that we were treated so well. But I am so old I changed my name when I got married. My father and I did not share a surname, and though some of the staff knew who I was, the engaging young man who came to collect the equipment from Home Loans certainly had not got a clue, and his smiling face, and considerable charm as he expressed his sympathies, were helpful in themselves. When I told him that the wheelchair had originally been delivered to my office and was now going back with him, and would he explain it to Cath, he looked at me quizzically and asked how I knew Cath. I explained I chaired the Trust, at which he seemed completely unfazed, and just said – correctly – that I did not look the same as I did in my photographs. That was not entirely surprising after three days and nights in the same pair of jeans, and going though a roller-coaster of emotions, plus exhaustion.

It was only a few weeks later that my father-in-law died at home, and was also looked after by some of our district nurses. There the name was the same as mine. But everyone by then knew that he was not my father. Once again, the care was remarkable. He had private nurses as well, and the integration between NHS and private worked extraordinarily well. The district nurses provided great comfort to my father-in-law, but also remark-

able support to my mother-in-law, husband, brother-in-law and the rest of the family. Once again, it was a faultless service. Once again, an elderly man died in his own home, surrounded by loved ones, pain-free and peacefully – as he, and his family, had wanted.

I know it is not always like this. I hear all too often of parts of the country, even parts of London, where such care is not made available, where the palliative care service does not cover weekends, or really provide a proper service integrated with the community nurses. But our experience was quite wonderful. It leaves us all with a feeling of deep gratitude, of wonder at the devotion of the people who provide that service day after day to very distressed people, and also quite certain that we should provide this for everybody, everywhere, throughout the country. The NHS has got this right. We ought to shout about it much more loudly, show it to other countries where people still die hospitalised, intubated deaths. But, first, we must make sure it is possible for everyone here in the UK to receive such care – because it feels absolutely right.

First Person, *Health Service Journal*, 3 October 1996. (reprinted with permission)

Five years later, my mother died. She had also been ill for a very long time, from before the time my father died, though we made light of her illness, telling her that it was my father who was ill. How unkind that seems now. She had a horrible auto-immune disease, manifesting itself in a variety of ways, including sudden total loss of hearing, painful legs, renal failure, odd skin lesions. Wegener's Disease, or, as she described it, the attentions of Mr Wegener, is a singularly unpleasant, unpredictable condition, with which she suffered considerably but also showed immense courage in the face of its worst onslaughts. Here follows the piece I wrote for *The Observer* at the time:

My mother died in May 2001, after four years of an auto-immune disease which left her with painful legs, poor kidney function, and general lassitude. There was little the doctors could do, but she went regularly to see her 'professor' at University College Hospital, argued about how much steroid she was prepared to take, and hoped for some miracle.

It never came, but injections of erythropoietin over those four years, by Breda Sheehan, her beloved district nurse, and regular visits from GP Jonathan Sheldon, made her illness more bearable, and alleviated the worst of the symptoms.

But from January of that year, it was clear she was deteriorating, and from mid-April we were into the last few weeks. At that point, the service we received was ratcheted up a few notches. After a fall, she was taken to the Royal Free Hospital. Despite their being on a 'take' for University College, my mother was treated with the utmost courtesy, visited by the care of the elderly team as well as the A&E Registrar, allowed to go home provided she was careful, and visited the following day by the specialist occupational therapists.

Two weeks later, with things obviously deteriorating, we moved to daily district nurse visits from Breda, to support not only my mother, but the devoted carers too.

Her GP came to talk to both my mother and me at my mother's flat, so that he could discuss with her what her worst fears were, allay them, plan for what might be needed, and set it up before he went on holiday. My mother was terrified of going into a home, of losing control. For someone who had been a refugee from Nazi Germany, security was important. Together, Jonathan Sheldon and I promised her she could stay at home. That is what she did.

A week later my mother had a major collapse. Melodie Francis, her palliative care nurse, and Breda were both there, and thought she was dying. We were called. By the time the afternoon came and went, my mother was sitting up in bed reading the paper. Breda, Melodie, my husband and I were all exhausted, and bemused. So it went for a few days, until we began the final decline.

At that point, Breda and her colleagues were visiting up to five times a day: my mother needed help with virtually everything, and one carer was not enough. Melodie was coming in two or three times a day, because my mother turned out to be allergic to morphine; she itched frantically, we scratched in sympathy. Pain control, particularly with the cramps she was then experiencing, was quite difficult. But controlled it was, and if it meant calling Breda out again, it was never too much trouble. If we needed help at night, it was there.

Towards the last, when we had been on an emotional roller-coaster, the team members turned their attention to all of us as well as their prime patient. Mrs Ryan, May, Juliet, Cavell, and Hayley, her 'team' of carers, were supported, as were her family. Breda joked with my children, who were facing university exams, teased my husband, comforted me, and helped to keep the atmosphere light and supportive. At the end, we had private night nurses for my mother, so that she could have pain relief whenever it was needed, and so that we could get some sleep. Once again, those nurses fitted brilliantly into the system.

My mother died as she wished, in her own home, compos mentis, surrounded by people she loved, and by her own things. She slipped away, in an NHS-provided hospital bed with an air mattress, with the best possible care anyone could have.

But that was not all. Within three days, the equipment, the drugs, the stuff needed for my mother's care had been removed by people whose condolences were genuine. Breda continued to come to see us, to make sure we were all right, and Melodie rang to check that I was coping.

I do not believe that the private sector on its own could ever deliver a *service like this, with the component parts working smoothly and apparently effortlessly together. I know that there is huge effort in making those partnerships work, but we experienced the result of that hard work in a magnificent service where organisational boundaries never showed. We saw the NHS at its best – across community services and the acute sector, across primary care and palliative care. And they worked happily with the private sector.*

At best, this country has services for people who are dying and their families which are incomparable. We should praise them more. Reading newspapers and watching television, one might think the NHS never gets it right. But what we have just experienced makes it clear that it can be superb. I am grateful for the way my mother's dying was supported, for it makes the pain of loss easier to bear.

More to the point, the real appreciation was hers. She thought she was wonderfully looked after, with remarkably little pain and distress. Before she died, she too blessed the NHS, and thanked her carers, her nurses, NHS and private, her GP, her consultants, and everyone else who had made dying like that possible. It was truly remarkable.

These articles give some flavour of what we experienced as a family, with the help of professionals who were both amazingly kind – in my view beyond the call of duty – and superbly professional and knowledgeable. Their skills, knowledge, and human warmth, were a real help and comfort to my family and my parents' friends – I do not believe either of my parents would have had such good deaths had it not been for those people. Equally, five years apart and two different teams, with different GPs and primary care teams involved, suggests that this is more of a pattern than isolated instances – and that from that pattern, and what those experiences teach us, we can learn much more about dying well. So, to those who made the going easier for both my parents, and to those who made their dying easier for all of us, this book is dedicated – to them, their skills, and their devotion.

How we can die well, and help our families, friends, patients and neighbours die well too.

Julia Neuberger
May 2004

Acknowledgements

This second edition is in memory of my parents, Walter and Liesel Schwab, and is dedicated to all those who made my parents' deaths easier, happier and better, supporting my family and me in May 1996 and again in May 2001, especially Ann Hamlet, David Evans, Tom Evans, Breda Sheehan, Jonathan Sheldon, Melody Francis, Nuala Ryan (snr) and Juliet Mwaniki.

1

An introduction to the history of ideas about death

Wherever we are in the world, whatever our age, our gender, our class, we all have feelings about death. Those feelings are often poorly expressed, even poorly acknowledged. For many peoples throughout the world, how they bury or cremate their dead, and how they mourn them, labels the group from which they come, the tribe. Often it says little about belief but far more about culture. Often it says little about individual desires but more about community expectations. How we view our deaths, how we treat our dying, how we console the bereaved, how we care for the carers, is universal subject matter. But how it is addressed varies considerably from individual to individual, from group to group, from country to country, from healthcare system to healthcare system, from you to me to her to him. There are no universal answers to the question: 'How will I, or you, or him, or her, meet the end?'

The idea of the good death is an ancient one. The Biblical expression of being gathered to one's fathers has a certain restfulness to it, and, indeed, an idea of what is normal. We are supposed to die in generational order, parents before children, grandparents before parents. We are supposed to be gathered to our fathers and mothers. The most satisfactory outcome to be desired is that we will die peacefully, possibly aware that we are near our end, having achieved most of what we wished to achieve. Our hope is that there will be no pain, either physical or emotional (a hope rarely completely achieved), and that we will either know nothing about it (dying at home in our sleep) or that we will know very little, just enough to say our farewells to those we love.

We would like to be like Abraham, in the Hebrew Bible:

And these are the days of the years of Abraham's life which he lived, an hundred threescore and fifteen years. Then Abraham gave up the ghost, and died in a good old age, an old man and full of years, and was gathered to his people. And his sons Isaac and Ishmael buried him in the cave of Machpelah, in the field of Ephron the son of Zohar the Hittite ... (Genesis 25:7–9) in the cave which Abraham had bought from Ephron as a burial place for his first wife, Sarah, and which became the family tomb.

Or, if we cannot be like that, and perhaps some of us might have our doubts about reaching the age of 175, worried about who will care for us, we would certainly like to be like Moses, who, though he did not go into the promised land, saw it from the top of Mount Nebo, and was:

an hundred and twenty years old when he died: his eye was not dim, nor was his natural force (sexual powers) abated. (Deuteronomy 34:7)

We would all like that. Or even to be like King David, who said to Solomon his son:

I go the way of all the earth (1 Kings 2:2)

and then gave him instructions:

Be thou strong therefore and shew thyself a man; and keep the charge of the Lord thy God, to walk in his ways, to keep his statutes, and his commandments, and his judgments, and his testimonies, as it is written in the law of Moses, that thou mayest prosper in all that thou doest, and whithersoever thou turnest thyself. (1 Kings 2:2–3)

These are only a few examples of the peaceful deaths we encounter reading though ancient Hebrew literature, though possibly – in the Greek classics at least – we read more about the violent deaths in battle, or in some kind of disgrace. As a result of the texts that are our legacy, we know about how suicide was abhorrent to many ancient peoples – yet there was a wholly acceptable form of martyrdom: killing the women and children before turning the swords on themselves, rather than falling into the hands of particular enemies. We know that city captors often treated their captives to cruel and prolonged deaths by torture. And, of course, we read about women dying in childbirth as well, a commonplace event. So the expressions about death we cherish are those of a peaceful death, being gathered to our ancestors, or 'sleeping' with them. The image of an endless rest is an appealing one. The idea that our rest might be broken in an afterlife, with torment as punishment for acts we have performed in this life, is a later idea, and a deeply disturbing one.

Yet the idea of an underworld, peopled by demons and guards, is itself an ancient one. The ancient Greeks and Romans believed in their underworld, with Charon the boatman taking the dead across the Styx to Hades, where a shadowy existence continued. Ancient Greek funeral customs included putting a coin in the mouth of the deceased person as they were being prepared for burial, in order that they had the money to pay Charon for the fare across the river. And bodies had to be buried quickly – not, as many have argued, because of the heat of the summers in the ancient world, but to prevent the spirit wandering about aimlessly – presumably because it was thought that just such an aimless spirit could do damage if it decided to do so. It was Christianity that developed the idea of Heaven and Hell, as well as Purgatory, possibly out of older ideas about the underworld, and with other influences at work such as Mithraism, a religion that was enormously popular in the Roman world. Judaism was later in its construction of an idea of a place for an afterlife. Whilst the place to which the dead go in the Hebrew Bible is Sheol, the pit, a belief grew up in rabbinic Judaism, very likely under Christian influence, or in competition with the successful prosely-tising of Christianity, in Heaven, in a place to which we go (often named pardes, i.e. Paradise). The idea of punishment and reward grew, and it stretched out through Christianity and Islam as well, especially the reward or punishment of the soul, as distinct from the body, immediately after the death. The idea of the resurrection of the dead at the end of days began to grow too, a concept not found in the Hebrew Bible except in the extraor-dinary prophecies of the prophet Ezekiel, in his vision about the valley of dry bones:

> And he said to me, Son of Man, can these bones live? And I answered, O Lord God, thou knowest ... And when I beheld, lo, the sinews and the flesh came up upon them, and the skin covered them above; but there was no breath in them ... And ye shall know that I am the Lord, when I have opened your graves, O my people, and brought you up out of your graves. (Ezekiel 37:3,8,13)

The fascination with death, and with the possible future life of the dead, is an ancient one. One has only to look at Egyptian tomb paintings, and to learn a little about the ancient Egyptian obsession with death, and the world of the dead, to the extent that the dead person took everything necessary with them to the next world, servants, meals, clothes, and so on, to realise that the next world was as 'real' to them as this. Concepts of Heaven in many traditions are very similar to the ideal life as lived on earth, too, and Egyptians are not alone in packing up everything someone might need for them to take with them on their journey to the afterlife. We see it dramatically in Chinese customs, as well as in what we read in Homer of the death of Patroclus and the human sacrifice that took place at the time. Equally, there is some pretty unpleasant evidence of what the Vikings did in the ninth and tenth centuries, when burying one of their hero warriors. A slave-girl, of no status, would be forced to have sex with a selection of the chieftains, and would then be ritually murdered and buried with the deceased hero. And there is much more – all of these customs suggesting that something had to be done to give safe passage to wherever the dead person was going, something to give help – it could be pots and pans, a concubine, servants, money or such like. The Aztecs forced their prisoners to be buried alive – or killed them first – in their funeral rituals for their dead heroes, and in Bronze Age Nitriansky Hradok, in modern Slovakia, there were 10 apparently praying, kneeling individuals buried alive – willingly, according to some authorities, though Timothy Taylor (2002) suggests that willingness is a curious term to use of those who might have felt duty, altruism or fear for their own afterlives or, even, the present lives of their children and families. We do not know. Suffice it to say that the ancient world seems to have many examples of human sacrifice as part of death rituals for those who have died naturally or in battle, and that the idea of taking people with you in death to the next world was commonplace.

Along with all that, there were the prayers and rituals needed for the dead person to get to where they needed to be. Indeed, the depiction of the sun god, Ra, making his journey by boat across the sky and then going under the earth to the world below – some equivalent to the world of the dead – and being reborn every day shows a little of the thinking behind Egyptian concepts of the world beyond this life. It is, of course, a universal human concern, as is fear of death, fear of pain, and a way of looking at one's end without being able simply to accept it and ignore it. For human beings, however matter-of-fact, there is too much emotion associated with our end, even where life is cheap, and where grief seems to modern western people either too short-lived or overly ritualised.

There is also the feeling that 'we shall meet again', a feeling shared by people who are dying and people who are bereaved, something that has its ancient origins in the idea of an afterlife where all will gather, or in the ideas about a final resurrection at the end of days when everyone will be resurrected at their best, and meet again. But the sense that people who have been separated in death will meet again is very strong in many cultures and religions, including Britain where formal religion has been in considerable decline for many decades.

More recent thinking about death

In modern times, in the west, ideas about the good death originate very largely from the 18th century. The good death was pain free, or pain dulled by laudanum. It consisted in saying one's goodbyes surrounded by one's family. The later, overly sentimental, Victorian pictures of deathbed scenes actually originate from the 18th century concept of the good death, where farewells were said, where prayers were said, where the family came to say goodbye, and where death itself was not a terrifying presence.

The anticipation of a good 18th century person was of a moment to say goodbye at death. 'Ars moriendi', the art of dying, is, amongst other things, the title of a medieval treatise that contains images of horrible and persuasive demons who prey upon a person's last moments, and which necessitate a firm hold on Christian belief in order to counter them. But the idea of an art in dying, the art of dying well, is probably as old as humanity itself, and the problem that has hit us in the 20th and 21st centuries is that, from the end of the Victorian era on, we have used euphemisms for death, regarded those who discuss death as morbid, and somehow forgotten that the experience of dying is as important as almost any other experience for human beings, and deserves proper consideration, though not obsession.

It is worth thinking about our use of langauge for a moment. All too often, we do not even say that someone has died. We say instead that they have 'passed on' or 'passed away'. They are 'the dear departed', or the 'one who has gone to his/her eternal home'. Euphemisms came into common usage in the Victorian age, but that was a time when death was, if anything, overly marked. The Victorians took the funeral and grief to hitherto unknown degrees of observance; some would argue that many Victorians themselves became obsessional, including Queen Victoria in her profound grief for Prince Albert. Whatever the truth of that, it is at the end of the Victorian age that the plethora of euphemisms really hit the English scene. Non-conformists seem to have been the first to use them, but it became commonplace soon after, so that when George V died in 1936, his death was announced on BBC radio as the fact that he 'had passed peacefully away'. The word death was not used. People 'passed away', 'fell asleep', 'departed this life'. In military action, they 'copped it', or 'their number was up'. And colloquialisms abound – people 'pop their clogs', 'hop the twig', and 'turn their toes up'. There are many more such expressions.

But, if these are the expressions that are used, if saying the word 'death' becomes less common, even less acceptable, the idea that one might contemplate one's death, as early religious thinkers would have urged us to do, would have seemed morbid. Indeed, the consideration of death and dying at all was considered morbid during the middle of this century – which did not stop people studying and talking about the subject. But it was not a subject for polite society. When Ian Crichton wrote his book, *The Art of Dying*, which was published in 1976, he started with the fact that everyone had told him it was a morbid subject when they had asked what he was writing about and he had told them. When Sarah Boston and Rachel Trezise were working on their TV series and book for Channel Four, *Merely Mortal*, a decade later, they were met with the same reaction. Indeed, approaching terminally ill patients for discussions with them for the film was an exercise in tact itself, given the sensitivities.

How then, with these attitudes so prevalent in our time, can one talk properly about the good death? How can this be done, particularly in the light of the fact that either we are considered morbid to want to talk about it

at all, or we are drawn away from it in embarrassment because of the awareness of how many people have been killed violently, in war, genocide, or by
famine and suffering, who had no chance to think about a good death in
reasonable old age? And did that reluctance to discuss death hit us in the
wake of the First World War, when so many young men were killed in the
trenches, when barely a family in Britain was untouched by loss? Was death
the great unmentionable, the stuff of nightmares and panic attacks but not of
debate and discussion and comfort? For, though from the 16th century on,
people had kept a 'memento mori' – a picture of a skull and a Bible, just a
skull or some other reminder by their side – to remember that we must die,
from the end of the First World War onwards that custom became deeply
unfashionable. We did not want to remember that we must die. Too many
had just died, before their time, and those that had returned had their nerves
shot to pieces, and were blinded or aimless and deeply depressed. Hence the
lack of discussion, and hence the reaction of the 1970s and 1980s to an
unmentionable subject – now once again fashionable, but still too rarely made
unemotional, factual and practical.

Yet, during all this period, some have continued to think about it, and write
about it. In some ways, discussion of some aspects of death and dying has
become fashionable, particularly some of the details surrounding physical
relief of pain and the attendant emotional, and psychological, relief that goes
along with it, allowing a different kind of contemplation. The old adage, that
we should live every day as if it were our last, or that we should repent one
day before we die – on the basis that it should be a permanent state, for most
of us cannot know exactly when we will die (Mishnah: Ethics of the Fathers
II:15) – has somehow stuck with us. You cannot ignore it. Though various
studies have shown people shying away from it (quoted by John Hinton in
his superb book *Dying*), the majority of people have wanted to think about it
and talk about it, as TV programmes on euthanasia, and on the ever-popular
hospice movement, make abundantly clear.

Indeed, the hospice movement, which has so caught the imagination of the
British public that it has become one of the most popular human charities,
expresses the desire people have for a 'dignified death', an expression one
hears all too often, and which, even with the best will in the world and the
best offices of the hospice movement and other palliative care services, is
unlikely to happen. Death is not a dignified business, in most cases, though
that does not militate against us dying well, even enjoying, odd though that
may read, 'a good death'.

In some extraordinary way, the 19th century, particularly the latter half of
it, destroyed that concept of the good death. The Victorians were wonderful
at funerals and at mourning. All the rules about purple and black, about large
funerals, about great new cemeteries that were monuments to magnificent
architecture and stonemasonry, are Victorian. Exhibitions on the subject of the
Victorian way of death show all too clearly how they rejoiced in a funeral
train to go to Randall's Park at Leatherhead in Surrey, or how the great

monuments of the south London cemeteries came to be constructed. A decent funeral came to be every working person's desire and dream. Until the 1940s and even later in some parts of the British Isles, people were putting away a shilling a week for their funerals, giving it to the insurance man when he came round. My mother, when she first came to Britain from Nazi Germany as a refugee, had never encountered the shilling for the funeral before. But amongst working girls at Marks and Spencer in the 1930s, it was still commonplace. Decency in death was as important, possibly even more important, than decency in life.

But it became overly sentimentalised, in two distinct ways. First, there was the sentimentality surrounding the death of children. Sunday school prize novel after Sunday school prize novel told the tale of an angelic child, often, but not always, female, who was going to Heaven. We saw her in a golden glow, with fair hair shining. The child was saying goodbye to her not too grief stricken family, who knew she was on her way to a better place. The best known picture of a doctor attending a dying child, Sir Luke Fildes' *The Doctor*, where a child lies dying with the doctor beside her in a fisherman's cottage on the English coast, uses that particular theme, that particular lie, one might almost add. There are thousands upon thousands of stories like that to be found in second-hand bookshops, but the style of thinking about a child's death is by no means original in those volumes. For the classic of all times in that regard is perhaps Charlotte Brontë's *Jane Eyre*, where, towards the beginning of the schooldays at the appalling Lowood school, a real school which Charlotte Brontë both attended as a child and where she later taught, Helen Burns dies of consumption. Helen was almost certainly Charlotte's own sister Maria, and the conversation which Helen and the young Jane have is one which both reduces the reader to tears and irritates beyond measure. For Helen herself is sure she is going to a better place. There will be no more earthly pain. Jane is not to grieve for her too much. As I have got older I have felt more and more angry about that idea that Jane should not grieve for her too much. 'Why not?', I hear myself asking. The need to grieve is a very human one. To somehow find solace in the idea that the dear departed has gone to a better place is one thing, but not to be allowed to grieve because of it seems extraordinary, when the grief is largely to do with missing the person, and having terrible feelings of disappointment at what they failed to achieve in their life because it was cut short. And, in this case, the fictionalised person whose life was cut short was the author's sister, a child who died unnecessarily because conditions at the school were so appalling.

But *Jane Eyre* takes the sentimentalising of childhood deaths to its apogee, possibly as a literary device to pour scorn on the school and its governors who allowed such conditions which led to the girls' illnesses and deaths to persist. There are thousands of examples, however, and the Victorian imagination on the subject of childhood death, at a time when the death of children was common, is one that still colours some of our thinking, even though we now find the death of children in the west virtually unbearable.

But the other important factor in Victorian thinking about death, at least within the English speaking world, was the death of Queen Victoria's husband, Prince Albert, and her lifetime of mourning for him. She took mourning to a fine art herself. She insisted on court mourning, on great memorials, including the vast Albert Memorial in Hyde Park. And she barely came out of her mourning to celebrate any event at all after his death. That, in itself, had a powerful impact on the public, and set an example of how we should approach death, with formality, and outward visible signs of mourning, and with memorials and black-edged cards, and black-edged newspapers, and so on. So black became the colour favoured by widows in Victorian England (it had always been the colour of mourning in the Mediterranean countries) and the commonplace stationery of grief became black cards and black-edged envelopes, to be bought cheaply at any stationers. Black for mourning. Pink and gold for the colours of expectation of heaven, particularly for children. That was done in books, at least in part as a result of the thinking that, for many of the children who died in appalling conditions of poverty and disease, the fact was that their lives had been 'nasty, brutish, and short'. Heaven for innocent children had to be better than that. Though whether this was simply a way of coping with commonplace child death is unclear – it may well be that conditions looked so appalling for so many of those children that anything would seem a release from the objectionable. Yet the sentimentalisation of childhood death must have slowed quite considerably the effect of the anger of those social reformers who looked at conditions and saw how dramatically and how speedily they could be improved. Indeed, with the rise of the 'respectable' working classes, the assumption was that decent conditions could be found in poor homes if they tried hard enough – and the working classes themselves went along with these major mourning rituals, with the wearing of black, and with the invention of that new sign of mourning, the black armband.

But the Victorian fascination with death, and almost celebration of it, changed with the coming of the new century. With telegraph and the telephone, it became possible to hear news of death in war all too quickly. The savagery of the First World War and the needless loss of life, the sense that thousands of young men had died quite unnecessarily in the trenches, was one element in a changing attitude towards death. Death in war, death before one's proper time, death of the prize of England's youth, the agony of the war poets, all this added up to a different attitude. Much of that has been recorded in the writing of the time and later – no-one can fail to be moved by Pat Barker's evocation of the smell of death in her Booker prize winning *The Ghost Road*, or by the pain recorded in Vera Britain's *Testament of Youth*, as the flower of England's youth met its end. Death was painful. It had to be faced, by almost every family with young men serving in the army. But it was no longer sentimental. A much darker tone hit descriptions of death. Blood, mud and gore were featured. Wilfrid Owen captured a mood of despair. The trenches were about fear, and stenches, and rats. Young men who survived returned with nightmares, often politely described as 'shellshock'. It was not the shells that had shocked them. They had seen their friends and comrades die. They kept reliving their experiences. Psychological interventions were in their infancy. Yet these young men could no more 'pull themselves together' than fly. The spectre of death in its worst guises kept returning to haunt them. Victorian sentimentality would no longer do. So descriptions of death darken, and then they gradually disappear. After the First World War poets, death as a theme becomes less common. Instead, with Freudian thought capturing the world, people began to talk about sex (long before the 1960s).

Yet, as ordinary talk of death disappeared in the main from literature, a movement for birth control for the working classes, and for euthanasia for the unfit, was beginning. Eugenics was growing in popularity, and had its darker side. For instance, long before the Nazi programme of extermination of the Jews, the early Nazi policy makers came up with the idea of exterminating all those who were living in state institutions who were mentally ill or handicapped, on cost grounds. The most extraordinary piece of deceit took place. Whilst parents were being told of their children's new clothes, and that they were eating well, their children were being systematically murdered, with the connivance of churchmen, very often – though it was church objections that finally halted the process – and all this was with the active participation of psychiatrists, who had been unable to help the young men returning from the First World War trenches.[1] It took a long time for the German psychiatric profession to retrieve its professional standing after that. But it also helps to explain, even before the mass exterminations of Jews, gypsies and others, why the view of death changed from one of sentimentalisation to one of horror – brutal war, brutal extermination, the beginnings of a scientific theory about the survival of the fittest being used to justify murdering the less fit.

And then there was the Holocaust, and the systematic murder of millions of civilians, quite apart from the other casualties of the Second World War. People who had lived through the death camps could not talk about them. Others were filled with horror of death. All this deliberately engineered death was happening just at the time that it was increasingly possible to keep people alive. The old-time deaths from tuberculosis were slowing down with the discovery of antibiotics. Polio was gradually disappearing with inoculation and vaccinations for other childhood diseases were making their mark. Life expectancy was shooting up. Normal death at a young age was becoming less common. Abnormal death at a young age was much to be feared. And people did not talk.

Only in some of the new West Indian communities of the 1950s and 1960s in Britain, the Windrush generation and its successors, was there discussion of death, and a more open way of marking dying and bereavement. In West Indian communities, deathbed scenes were commonplace – and often still are – and the churches supported both the dying people and their families, with a huge funeral in many cases, and rituals that recognised the importance of grief as well as a sense of joy in the expectation of a very real Heaven.

A modern reflection

But, apart from very specific communities with a different view, in main-stream Britain, by the time I was growing up in the 1950s and 1960s, my generation was not familiar with dead bodies. I did not see a dead body until I was in my twenties. As genocides became more common – Cambodia, Rwanda, Uganda, to name but a few – most of my contemporaries were the same. They had never seen a dead body, except on television, in appalling images of large numbers of corpses. But they were not real to them in most cases. More than never having seen a dead body, they probably had not been to a funeral. For many of them, the first funeral they went to was that of a parent or grandparent. Ordinary death, ordinary people dying ordinary deaths at home surrounded by their loved ones, was disappearing. People we knew died in hospital. It was somehow more hygienic. You did not have to think about it; or see it; or be there. It would all be tidied away. Just as babies began to be born in hospital as the norm, so people began to die in hospital. It was the norm and we all accepted it. We did not talk about death. We did not draw down the curtains when the cortège went past for the funeral, unless we lived in Scotland or Ireland. We simply ignored it, despite increasing news of people starving, or being killed in appalling regional wars, and growing genocidal killings.

Meanwhile, those who died in hospital had a less than easy time of it as well. Hospitals were places for curing people, not for looking after them when they were dying. All the training of young doctors and nurses was geared towards getting people better, not to alleviating their pain and discomfort when they could no longer improve. Patients who were dying were all too often shoved into a side ward, given a massive dose of morphine every four hours, and left to get on with it. Little was done to alleviate their distress. All too little was understood about their pain, physical and mental, and though cruelty was not intended, it took place every day.

For, to be packed away and left to die alone, in pain, is a terrible experi-ence for anyone. In a culture where no-one was even talking about death any more, it was cruel. The dying people were often not even told that that is what they were doing. They were given false reassurances in blustery, jolly voices: 'Oh, you'll soon be out of here...' (In a box...!) 'We'll get you up and about in a jiffy...!' (Not bloody likely.) But the prevailing attitude was not to talk. So the dying person would lie there, high as a kite on morphine for a couple of hours, and in pain, disorientated, without anyone to tell him or her honestly what was happening, with a few people coming in from time to time to talk about the weather – but nothing that mattered.

To some extent, this remains the case, but such practice is diminishing. Yet, even now, all too often, where a person cannot die in a hospice or at home, staff in hospitals or in nursing homes, unintentionally, treat dying patients in a cavalier way. In many cases, they have not been trained to do otherwise.

The ethos of many teaching hospitals is, in any case, to go for acute intervention rather than skilled care of people who in some sense have 'no hope' in the terms of cure-motivated health professionals. Indeed, it is further complicated by the fact that people with very little chance of recovery or even of remission and survival for any length of time worth talking about, are subjected to heroic interventions, which may be more for the benefit of the carers than of the patients. If carers themselves, healthcare professionals, have been brought up like the rest of us, then unless they have been trained specially, they will be unfamiliar with death. Even now in hospitals, they may regard it as their duty to try to avert death rather than welcome it, making the patient comfortable in the process.

This has reached a far more serious stage in the United States than in Europe. For, in the USA, there is almost an attitude that death is to be averted in all possible circumstances, that there is no natural lifespan. Life expectancy after the age of 84 is higher than in the rest of the western world. People lie in intensive care for months, with battle being waged against death. And so people die horrible, prolonged, intubated deaths, well recorded by Sherwin Nuland in his year-long 1994 US best-seller, *How We Die*. But what he describes, and what we can see in the wards of American hospitals, cannot be the kindest way to go.

It is as a result of this kind of thinking, this desire to preserve life, that a new movement grew up in the 1980s and 1990s for people to sign a living will, an advance directive, in the United States. Indeed, as a result of legislation passed in 1991 (The Patient Self-Determination Act), every institution in receipt of state or federal funds, which means more or less everywhere in the American healthcare system, has to ask a patient each time they are admitted whether or not they have signed an advance directive or appointed a healthcare proxy. Although many institutions have not taken this altogether seriously, to the extent that they have allowed the cleaning staff to ask the question, on the grounds that everyone else is too busy, the intention behind the legislation is altogether clear. Patients should be able to decide for themselves when they want no more treatment. And they should be able to decide, in advance of being in a state where they cannot make their wishes known to their carers, as to what it is they want done, or not done. Of course, this is in part a reaction against the worst excesses of the American healthcare system, with people being kept in intensive care for months, full of tubes, unable to tell night from day. But it is also a form of rationing – it is an attempt to cut down the absolutely huge sums of money spent on patients in the last few weeks of life. Indeed, there are those who argue that half of all health expenditure is spent in the last six months of life. The thinking surely goes like this: If people can make advance directives, they will decide to have less expensive, less interventionist treatment if they are mentally unfit, and will therefore spend less on care, which will in turn cost the state or the federal government less. But there is disturbing evidence from the *New England Journal of Medicine* that one in four advance directives has been disregarded.[3] Nevertheless, the thinking is about treating those who are very ill, and probably dying, more humanely, or at least more in accord with their own wishes.

Questions of conscience

For this is really the problem. From the late 20th century onwards, we have had choices about how we die if we live in the western world – with its extra-ordinary healthcare that can often keep us alive, if not living. We can make choices about how hard to try to stay alive, about whether to go for pain control and comfort, or heroic, but unlikely, interventions. Yet, even the unlikely interventions sometimes work. Many of us have things we still want to do, still want to achieve, or see happen. There is a possibility that we might be able to get some of those things done, if we submit ourselves to some of the interventions that are sometimes suggested, unpleasant though they might be. Do we have to have the treatment every time? Can we say to ourselves we have had enough? These are questions of conscience for each of us as individuals now, but they are also questions of conscience for every healthcare professional. Should the doctor or the nurse decide who should live, and for how long, or not? Whose decision should it be, now we can take it, whether to go for life-support? The doctor's? The nurse's? The patient's? The patient's family?

And how do we come to these decisions? Alone? With help? With that modern answer to all communications issues, a video? Watching a video alone? Is it my decision, or yours? Is it my body? Whose body is it anyway? And, once the decision is taken, should we then be able to say that we want complete pain relief, and to be put out of our misery if we suffer pain? And, if that is the case, does that justify us asking a doctor to kill us? For eutha-nasia is not legal in the United Kingdom, though it has been decriminalised in Holland. But discussions about its introduction are increasingly common, with Joel Joffe leading a campaign for its introduction in the House of Lords, and a committee being set up to examine it again in 2004. Meanwhile, the UK government is proposing legislation to allow advance directives in the UK (proposed for 2004), which will, at least, make it plain that choice of treatment is the dying person's choice, rather than the healthcare professionals'. And that has become ever more necessary as more and more cases are tested in the UK courts over whether someone has a right to die (the totally paralysed Miss B convinced judges she should be allowed to die, with a cessation of life preserving treatment, in 2002) or even whether they have a right to live, as cases are being tested at present (2004) over severely disabled Child N, whom healthcare professionals have, arguably, decided not to resuscitate when she has severe breathing problems. Or David Glass, the child whose disabilities led to doctors ceasing feeding and giving him a diamorphine drip at aged 11, on the basis that his severe disabilities made resuscitation absurd. His relatives unplugged the drip (*The Observer*, 4 January 2004) and resuscitated him themselves, and a ruling on what the law should be in these cases is expected from the European Court in early 2004. All these are cases which illustrate the difficulty. The question is whose control matters, and who gets to make the decision. In modern Britain, we increasingly seem to think that it is our choice, the dying person's and their family, the disabled person's and their family, and not for heath professionals. All this can be predicated, arguably, on a basic human right to control our own fate.

But how do we make those decisions sensibly, when circumstances have changed so much? For, alongside the development of techniques for keeping people alive, with the great advances in clinical medicine, goes the development of the modern hospice movement. Founded in Britain by Dame Cicely Saunders, OM, it has had a profound effect worldwide. For the modern hospice movement preaches pain control at the very beginning, and then caring for the whole person, not just the physical symptoms. It preaches care, and love, and faith. For those without faith, its philosophy can be hard to take. For those who prefer to think of themselves as autonomous individuals with the right to take their own lives, or ask others to take it for them, the hospice is curiously fatalistic. They prefer more decisive action, less prayer and faith. But for many people who do not share the intensity of Christian faith which Dame Cicely Saunders has, as do many of those working in the hospice movement, there is nevertheless much to be gained out of the skilled control of pain developed by the hospice movement, with the proper use of morphine and other drugs, in no greater quantities, indeed often smaller, than conventional hospitals. Yet the philosophy is of relief of pain, and allowing the person to go smoothly and painlessly into death.

The hospice movement has had a powerful impact. But it is by no means enough. Still fewer than 10% of people die in hospices. More now die at home, around 50%, and many of them with home care teams helping and supporting them and their carers. Even then, care is still infinitely better for those dying from cancer, AIDS or motor neurone disease than for those dying of congestive heart failure, for instance, or end stage renal failure. The hospice movement has done much to change our attitudes to dying, but its main focus has been on cancer, whilst many, older people particularly, die of other conditions and combinations of causes which the palliative care specialists have often ignored. So, far more still needs to be done to challenge the hi-tech view of death, the way that heroic interventions are carried out often for the benefit of the healthcare professionals, and the way caring for dying people in a regular hospital is often so disappointing. The task facing all healthcare professionals when dealing with dying people is to try to come to terms with the fact that many people do not want all the heroic efforts in the world, everything possible, in fact, to be done for them. They do, however, want to be made comfortable, and that, with the skills now available and the huge knowledge base about pain control which has been developed as a result of the hospice movement, is entirely possible. And they want dignity to the last. Meanwhile, some of us have the great good fortune, not necessarily regarded as such by our family and friends, to go to bed one night and simply not wake up, but we rarely talk about it as our hope. As one of my children put it when she was very young, to go to bed and wake up dead. For most of us, that is the ideal death. If there were to be just the smallest bit of warning, such as a hint a couple of weeks or months before, then we could be sure we had put our affairs in order, that we had done the best to sort out any mess we had left, and could die at peace. And dying at peace with oneself is something dying people often talk about as their most cherished aim.

How we die

But most of us do not die like that. We go to the doctor because we have an ache, a pain, a swelling in the breast or in the groin, or we are unable to pass water. We cannot eat or drink. We simply feel off colour. Or an ambulance is called because we have had a stroke, or a coronary attack, or a sub-arachnoid haemorrhage. One or other of these things is what gets most of us into the situation where we think we might have a terminal illness. Not all these conditions are by any means terminal. Our GP might laugh at us and say we are just imagining it. The breast lump turns out to be benign. The inability to pass water is just the usual prostate trouble without any malignancy. But we have had the fear. We have begun to worry. And nothing is quite the same afterwards, because the beginnings of worry stay in the backs of our mind. We have had our first intimations of mortality.

Then, for most of us, comes the real illness that lays us low, and turns out to be terminal. Often, we do not know that to be the case at the outset, and there are questions to be asked about the way we are treated when we have a life-threatening, but not necessarily terminal, illness. For the standard practice amongst healthcare professionals is to be less than wholly frank with the prognosis, on the basis that, if we knew how unlikely a cure, or a remission, was, we would be less likely to take the treatment. The situation is changing. In the United States, there may be little tact involved, but healthcare professionals tend to be more honest. In Britain, the younger doctors particularly are more inclined to give the full picture.

But it is not as simple as that. For giving the whole picture means different things to different people, at different times. If I were in my mid-forties, with two dependent children, and was told I had a life-threatening disease, I would be more likely, given my situation and my personality, to want to go for all the heroic interventions that might give me a bit more time. In my fifties, I begin to feel differently; less worried about my children now they are grown up, but with lots of things I still want to do in my life. I imagine, but, of course, cannot be sure, that if I were in my mid-seventies I would be more fatalistic (at precisely the time when the malignancy is likely to grow more slowly anyway) and decide against the very unpleasant forms of treatment in favour of perhaps fewer years or months of life. Yet again, some people in their mid-seventies would not take that view, and would regard the desire of healthcare professionals not to give the most heroic, and expensive of interventions, on the grounds of their age, as nothing short of discriminatory.

So, there are no easy answers. People vary considerably. They vary according to circumstances, age, education, faith and social class – and, most importantly of all, they vary according to their own personalities. Some people will be upbeat and positive, want to defeat this illness that has come upon them unawares, whilst others will be fatalistic, and simply say: 'Let God's will be done'.

But there comes a point, after that stage, when it becomes clear that the condition is terminal. It is vital, then, for healthcare staff to know how the individual reacted at the time it was thought that the condition might not be terminal at all, because on the basis of that knowledge it is easier to care for that person. If the individual was a fighter, he or she may continue to fight until the very end. It may make them harder to care for, but it is their good right to be like that, and it actually leaves many healthcare professionals, who have a similar belief in the importance of fighting for life, with a considerable respect for the individual. But the die is cast. The person is not going to get better. Indeed, the person is going to get worse, and die, in the reasonably near future.

Now the problems begin. First of all, the fact that they are going to die in 'the reasonably near future' means different things to different people. It could be a few days, or weeks, or months. But the urgency will take people differently, and medical staff are notoriously – and rightly – reluctant to put a time on what they think people have left, because it is so difficult to predict with any kind of accuracy at all.

The current situation

But as death becomes a subject it is easier to talk about and write about (and all the evidence points that way), then it should be easier to be honest. If that should be the case, it should be easier to have discussions about what people really want at the end of life, how they want to die, who they want around them, how the healthcare professionals can provide the best support, and, indeed, how the modern skills of life-preservation and of pain control can be used to greatest and most welcome effect.

When that comes about, we will have rehumanised, and, indeed, demedicalised, death. Death will happen in our homes, with us there holding the hands of our dying family members. It will happen in the presence of children. It will be considered as normal as it once was, not something one has to leave home to do. There will be expert professional help available, with Macmillan and other hospice home care nurses, with people who can give families a break, who know how to alleviate pain and discomfort, but they will come to the home. Or be available within a hospice setting, for not everyone can die at home, or will even want to, depending on the ability of their families to care for them. It will be a great tribute to the thinking behind the hospice movement, and the courage of many healthcare professionals, if that comes about. But, if we are to die well, we must be given the choice of dying at home, with support from professionals, without pain, and with our families around us. We must also be allowed to die our way, whatever that might be.

And for many healthcare professionals that is a concept difficult to grasp. But different cultures and religions have very different attitudes to how they wish to die, and to how they wish grief to be expressed, and those differences are important, and can make a huge difference to the well-being and comfort of individual patients. That knowledge, that ability to provide individuals with the death they want, within certain parameters, should enable us to have a good death, where and how we want it. It should also enable us to use the experience to show others there is nothing to fear. What we are doing is shedding this life, in a peaceful manner. No mysteries, no horror, no agony. Instead, a peaceful end, as we want it, in as conscious a partnership as possible with those who have been our life's companions and friends, supported by professional care provided by people with great skill in pain relief and emotional support.

References

1 Burleigh M (1994) *Death and Deliverance – Euthanasia in Germany 1900–1945.* Cambridge University Press, Cambridge.
2 Danis M, Southerland LI, Garrett JM *et al.* (1991) A prospective study of advance directives for life-sustaining care. *NEJM.* **324**: 882–8.

2

Grief – reactions normal and abnormal

When someone dies, we grieve. It is a natural human reaction, and we do it whether we are the person who is dying, who goes through a grieving process which is well-recorded and not entirely dissimilar to what those left behind experience, or if we are the ones who are bereaved. It is a process of extreme pain, with all kinds of attendant emotions – and there is no way out of it. One cannot, properly, not grieve after a death of a loved one, and emerge normal.

Literature is filled with accounts of grief, with people tearing out their hair, in ancient times cutting their flesh, pulling off their clothes, sitting in ashes and sackcloth, and so on. Grief, though not displayed openly on the stage as much as other great emotions, is displayed by Hamlet, by Lear, by Othello – all with complications, of course – as horrible, overwhelming, almost destroying (sometimes succeeding in doing so) the person who has been bereaved. It is perceived almost as a body blow, a shock to the system. But, despite dramatic renderings of grief, in real life it is still, often, something people are expected to keep hidden and private, when it is virtually impossible to do so.

How grief works and is put together has been explained fully by Dr Elisabeth Kubler-Ross, amongst others. In the 1960s she established a seminar at the University of Chicago to consider the implications of terminal illness for the patients and for those involved in their care. Her accounts of the attitudes which emerged during conversations and interviews are recorded in her book *On Death and Dying*, where she suggested that the stages through which someone is likely to pass in coming to terms with his or her own death are: Denial and Isolation; Anger; Bargaining; Depression; Acceptance, and (some have added) Hope. Kubler-Ross originally had acceptance not as a happy stage, but as one almost 'void of feeling', near the end, in her sequential unfolding of emotions. Other scholars and observers have tested Kubler-Ross's stages, and have some things to say about it. Colin Murray Parkes, the person who has perhaps most closely observed what people say and feel in Britain, has argued:

> Others might (and probably will) adopt a different terminology when describing the phases through which the dying person passes in the course of his illness. Since individual variation is so great, it is unlikely that any one conceptual system could be applied to all. (In his foreword to Kubler-Ross's On Death and Dying)

John Hinton, Lily Pincus and others have largely followed Kubler-Ross's description of the stages through which a person goes, but challenged the universal applicability of the stages, whilst recognising that there are stages which are observable and describable through which most dying people, and indeed bereaved people, go.

Michael Young and Lesley Cullen, in their excellent A Good Death: conversations with East Londoners, make the point that Kubler-Ross was studying patients in an institution. What she may have been observing, at least in part, was the effect of total institutionalisation, particularly for people who knew they were never going to emerge except in a coffin. As they say, denial, anger, bargaining, depression, acceptance, are precisely the way different people respond to incarceration in a total institution, leading to what Goffman terms mortification of the self.

Since people, increasingly, die in a hospice or at home, though there are still too many dying in hospital, those stages of experience of the total institution become much less relevant. There are also major differences between the reactions and experiences of the very elderly facing their own death and younger people, not to mention major differences according to community and religion.

It is not only the case with the experiences of those who are dying that there is such variation. Many people's grief also does not follow such a prescribed pattern. Nevertheless, 'stages' we can think about can help someone who is dying, and anyone in a caring role for them, to understand what is going on. It also helps explain our need for time and space in which to think, contemplate, explore loss, say goodbyes – and, therefore, is really helpful, both to those who are dying themselves, who want to think about how to do it well, and to those who are caring for them, particularly family or close friends.

There is a huge literature concerned with the processes of grief and mourning, much of it written to help our society re-learn how to deal with death, and to help people talk about it. Such literature helps those involved as carers, formal and informal, both to understand the nature and phases of 'normal' grief, and to be aware of abnormal grieving which may require specialist help. But it should not be forgotten that healthcare professionals providing care for the dying, however 'professional' and 'objective' their behaviour, cannot help but become involved with some of their patients. Indeed, they would not be human if they did not do so, and they are better nurses, doctors, physiotherapists and other professionals simply by virtue of their very human-ness. Thus, they too have to be allowed to grieve. And families of people who are dying have to help them to do so. I shall never forget, as a very young and inexperienced rabbi myself, visiting a ward at one of our local teaching hospitals, to find that the man I had come to visit had just died after several days of being cared for intensively by a very young nurse, who was 'specialling' him. She was distraught with grief, and had finally taken refuge in a linen cupboard to cry her eyes out, where the ward sister had found her and told her not to be so 'unprofessional'. I can only remember feeling that the sister concerned had got it all wrong, and that it was important that this young woman was expressing her grief over the death of an elderly man of whom she had become very fond.

Added to that, because of our strange attitudes to death in Britain, it is likely that that young woman had never sat with a dying person in her life before, so that, in addition to her very natural grief over the person concerned, she was experiencing something akin to shock. Her training should have included dealing with death, and her sister on the ward should have been sympathetic when she was upset – for it was a sign of a really caring nurse that she was upset at the death of 'her' patient. And it was entirely normal. But we often do not treat that reaction of initial grief as if it is normal at all.

Normal grief

Apart from Freud's early paper on mourning (1917), the first study to concentrate seriously on the management of acute grief as a definite syndrome with psychological and somatic symptomatology, was that of Erich Lindemann. In 1944 he published a paper, which argued that a clearly defined grief syndrome may appear immediately after a crisis, or may be delayed, or even, sometimes, apparently be absent. Grieving is a process of coping, which involves working at freeing oneself from total involvement in the loss of the person who has died, re-adjustment to the environment in which the dead person is no longer present, and forming new relationships, or establishing new ways of dealing with the old ones. Since Lindemann's work, others have made important contributions to our understanding of the processes of grief. The work Elisabeth Kubler-Ross carried out with dying people is perhaps the most familiar to a modern western audience, reaching far wider than the medical establishment. Colin Murray Parkes's studies of grief in adult life, published in 1972, cover similar ground on the basis of over 10 years' work with bereaved people. From within the psychoanalytic tradition, Lily Pincus published her partly theoretical and partly anecdotal book *Death and the Family* in 1976, and in 1977 Yorick Spiegel wrote *The Grief Process*. Spiegel's work is both practical and pastoral, bringing together psychotherapy, sociology, and theology.

Many people have written about death and dying since. Amongst those which are particularly useful as studies of grief are John Hinton's *Dying*, Rosemary Dinnage's anthology, *The Ruffian on The Stair*, and Peter Noll's remarkable study of himself, *In the Face of Death*. But people will find different volumes helpful at different times – this one merely hopes to pull out some of the main themes in grief brought about by death, either of the dying person, or of those near and dear to him or her.

Anger is the first reaction most of us have to the news of our impending death, even though we may have expected it, known in our heart of hearts that we were on the 'last lap', as it were. It is because of the anger that comes as a first reaction to the news that dishonesty often sets in within our family relationships, because the spouse who first heard about the impending death of a loved one, and experienced the anger, does not wish to get 'him any more upset, dear', or 'I cannot go through that ill-temper again, dear'. . . . But after the anger comes acceptance.

The stages are well-recorded, and have been known since the work of Colin Murray Parkes and others. Those stages of grief are the way grief is often expressed by the dying person, some of which is then mirrored in the grief that those who are bereaved experience after the death. But it is important that, when we – as the individual concerned or as the carer – are told about the prognosis, our spouse or family are told as well, or efforts are made to make sure that the individual does tell the family, because otherwise the nature of the anger is almost too much to bear.

As well as that, those who are looking after the individual or the family need to be aware that it may well not only be the individual who goes through the stages of disbelief, anger and acceptance, but also the spouse and the whole family. People close to a person who is dying do some of their grieving whilst they are still alive, and the ideal is if they can do it together. For the experience of grief is universal. It is a normal response to the loss of some significant person or object. Divorce, unemployment, the amputation of a limb are all examples of losses which can cause grief. For a dying person, all the losses come together at the same time, in the impending loss of his or her life, and the prospect of the loss of everything that means anything recognisable. We are also faced with the different aspect of the loss suffered in dying, which is, as is obvious, its finality.

Loss through bereavement is a crisis in which a person's whole previous equilibrium is upset. The normal responses are inadequate. The behaviour of bereaved people may become very unpredictable, and lead them to a sense of shame for the embarrassment they believe they cause. There can be a real loss of 'self'. In this crisis, various so-called 'phases' of grief are often evident. The processes are now well documented, with four main phases: numbness, shock, and partial disregard of the reality of the loss; a phase of yearning, with an urge to recover the lost object; a phase of disorganisation, despair, and gradual coming to terms with the reality of the loss; a phase of reorgani-sation and resolution. Though normal grief usually includes such phases, there is, of course, no universal way of providing help. Grief is a complex process; for some people it continues for a long time, or is never really completed, whilst for others it seems to progress gradually, without the need for any sort of intervention except for a sensitive listening ear on the part of our family and friends, and, of course, of any professional in regular contact.

The 'phases' of grief often overlap and are sometimes repeated in different ways and in different contexts. In CS Lewis's *A Grief Observed* (1961), his personal painful description of his own bereavement illustrates this:

Tonight all the hells of young grief have opened again; the mad words, the bitter resentment, the fluttering in the stomach, the nightmare unreality, the wallowed-in tears. For in grief nothing 'stays put'. One keeps on emerging from a phase, but it always recurs. Round and round. Everything repeats. Am I going in circles, or dare I hope I am on a spiral? But if a spiral, am I going up or down it?

In the play based on *A Grief Observed, Shadowlands,* and then the film, based on the story of Lewis's relationship as a confirmed bachelor with the woman, mother of two boys, who was to become his wife, there was relatively little play on the intensity of feeling between them in love, perhaps because he was such a confirmed bachelor, so averse to relationships with women. But when it came to the experience of parting through her terminal illness, the cruel cancer which destroyed her, then the picture of grief was a real and terrible one. It encompassed the emotional and the physical, the agonising pain of loss, the impossibility that he certainly felt in trying to comfort her sons, whose loss was perhaps even greater than his own. Such representations are important, for, better than words explaining the grieving process, they demonstrate it with no qualms about illustrating the intensity of pain, some-thing which theatre rarely manages to capture about the ordinary emotions (for grief is an ordinary, and normal, emotion or series of emotions, to go through).

Most care for bereaved people who are grieving is no longer the province of the clergy, since the role of the clergy has diminished so much, and so few of us are now religious believers in the true sense, at least amongst Christians. Clergy amongst Muslims, to some extent Jews, Hindus and Sikhs, still play a more significant role in this area. But as a result of the waning of mainstream Christian faith in Britain (significantly not in Ireland, north or south), much so-called 'pastoral care' comes better these days from the health professionals who are caring for the dying person in other ways. It then comes as part of the normal business, however distressing, of someone's death. One person is dying, and needs physical and emotional support. Another person is facing bereavement, and is trying to prepare for it whilst the dying person is still alive and demanding care. The professional carers, alongside family and friends, and working closely with them, are often best placed to give us support and to explain what is going on. The clergy often have a role with us as well, but often their role is secondary to the pastoral care of a healthcare team, for that team is willing and able to provide the whole gamut of care, and to provide emotional and physical support to a dying person and his or her family. Increasingly, hospital chaplains find themselves providing support to the healthcare team more than to individual patients, whose pastoral needs are being met outside, and by the healthcare professionals.

But it is nevertheless true that, at each phase of the grieving process, a pastoral figure – counsellor, priest, rabbi or whoever – can in some ways facilitate the grieving experience for us, by being aware of what is happening to us and sometimes interpreting it to us, or to the team who are looking after us. Sometimes, too, where there is a relationship with the clergyperson, he or she can help enormously over the stages of normal grief by 'being there' as a resource and point of reference while all our previous assumptions are being challenged and changed. Any clergyperson, along with any health professional, knows it is important to work at the bereaved person's own pace, allowing time for reminiscence, allowing space for anger. Our family and friends often have to be helped to see this, and to value time and space, wherever they can be found, for exploring some of the emotions so necessary to go through. For grief can neither be rushed, nor denied.

Those of us who help bereaved people may need to do such things as giving permission to weep, or simply saying that a particular reaction – of anger, resentment, loneliness, relief – is entirely normal. For, usually, it is. And people who are dying and those who are about to be bereaved, or have been, need reassurance, need to understand, that what we are going through, albeit horrible, is entirely normal. Whatever is needed in the way of pastoral care for the bereaved, the vital thing for all of us – patients, their carers, family and friends, healthcare professionals, clergy – is to realise we can never get it wholly right. We can only get it less wrong. Grief is painful. It is lonely, soul-destroying, difficult, depressing. What we can do is support people though the normal stages of their grief, encourage them with the thought that they are not alone, and nurse them into a more normal life, usually a year or so after the bereavement. But we do it because we want to provide care. It is for that reason that this section is included here in the book.

Abnormal grief

What has been described above is within the broadest of descriptions, 'normal'. But, at each phase of grief, things can go wrong. After the initial shock and numbness, when feelings begin to emerge, they are often expressions of protest, often tears or bouts of uncontrollable weeping, considered rather hysterical and un-English in many circles. These are, however, appropriate and normal expressions, though they may sometimes be suppressed and true feelings denied. If that happens, all too often various abnormal reactions may follow. For some there can be a 'super-spirituality', based on the idea that to acknowledge grief must be a sign of unbelief. After all, the deceased is going to a better place. One should be pleased for them. Obviously that is not felt by many people of a variety of different faiths or of none. But for some Christians it is fundamental, and in some sects, as only too well expressed in Jeannette Winterson's classic novel about fundamentalist Christianity, *Oranges are not the Only Fruit*, expectation of glory is considerable, rendering normal grief theoretically unnecessary, a complete denial of what it means to be human.

There is also, reasonably frequently, a tendency to overactivity which avoids facing the reality of the death. Death may be denied by 'mummifying' the deceased's room or belongings, which is why those of us providing any kind of care should argue for clearing up some of the dead person's possessions to take place as soon as possible. The normal weeping over a pair of shoes, or a much disliked jacket, can be very therapeutic. In some people there may be a strong temptation to 'contact' the deceased through spiritualism – the ouija board is a well-known phenomenon, and I have been appalled at the number of apparently normal, intelligent people I have known who have lost a parent, particularly, and tried to contact them through some kind of medium or spiritual method.

Anger which is not acknowledged and, therefore, does not resolve, is another problem. It can be projected on to carers, the priest or rabbi or imam, the doctor, the nurses, or the hospital. Another phenomenon of abnormal grief can be the normal depression, associated with the phase of yearning or despair, developing into a chronic depressive illness, associated with overwhelming feelings of guilt, for everyone feels guilty when bereaved. None of us ever succeeds in doing enough for the dying person however dearly we loved them. The guilt remains, for we cannot tell them we meant it to be different, we wanted it to be different. Abnormal grief allows that guilt, and that regret, to become so enormous as to overwhelm us, and that phenomenon often needs specialist help.

The later phase of acceptance, of gradually coming to terms with the loss, can be delayed or stopped altogether by someone who is bereaved withdrawing from friends and family. Bereaved people – particularly, but not only, widowed elderly people who have problems in getting out of the house anyway – can, and often do, become reclusive. Alternatively, the grieving person can become over-dependent on others and develop a hopeless, irresponsible helplessness. If any of these reactions become chronic, the proper resolution of grief may not be reached without skilled intervention, and the bereaved person will stay feeling alone and in the dark, instead of gradually, albeit very slowly after 50 years or more of marriage to the same dear person, emerging into normal life with the rest of us.

When things go wrong

On the whole, grief has to be understood as a family experience. For, too often otherwise, family and friends pretend that the death has somehow not occurred. That comes of embarrassment in the face of death. But that very embarrassment, the fact that people do find it difficult to talk about, makes it vital that they should. It also makes it clear, when they do not, that the bereaved person is going to be left alone in a loneliness hard to envisage unless one has been through it. For the loneliness becomes a world of make-believe. Family and friends will keep their distance, ostensibly to allow the bereaved person to grieve, but actually because they do not know what to say. Embarrassment, not cruelty, leads to the habit of leaving the bereaved person alone. But, though cruelty may not be the motive, the effect is most certainly cruel. It is better for us to say nothing but at least to be there and hold a hand, than to pretend that there is nothing to say and that the bereaved person needs 'time alone' to 'get over' their grief. Out of our own fear of death, or in order to avoid hurting the feelings of a dying relative, families have sometimes failed to give honest support while our loved one dies alone, or experiences grief alone, in great pain.

Loss through bereavement, especially loss of a marriage partner, is a major change, not only in the bereaved person's 'inner world', but also in all the external relationships of which we are a part. How people experience and handle loss will be affected by our own emotional histories and, often, by the extent to which our early experiences have affected our ability to cope with loss. If there are previous unresolved losses in our lives, bereavement may be a time when these earlier pains resurface. John Bowlby (1974) stresses how the experiences of 'attachment and loss' in early childhood, and the need for the growing child to cope with 'separation anxiety', are the main keys to understanding the processes of mourning. Earlier, Melanie Klein (1940) wrote about pain being necessary to renew the links to the external world and, thus, continuously re-experience the loss as well as rebuilding with anguish the inner world, which is felt to be in danger of deteriorating and collapsing.

When things go right

To those of us caring for the family, in which each person experiences their own grief as well as sharing in the grief of each other, Parkes (1972) suggests that something can be done to ease the pain. Amongst other ideas, he argues that much pain can be prevented if a person about to be bereaved can be encouraged to express some grief in anticipation, something health professionals can surely take on board, especially nurses who are caring for someone at the end or very near it. Secondly, a willingness to share the grief needs to be expressed by carers, though it should not be forced. Thirdly, carers have to realise that they cannot give the bereaved person what they really want, which is their beloved person back again – and the bereaved have to realise that carers and people providing pastoral care can only do a little to help. Fourthly, wider family and friends can do a great deal to cushion the blow – their presence really does help in many cases, even if it does so by what some Jews would call an 'aggravation factor'. So irritated can we, as bereaved people, become with an enormous number of relatives being around, trying to be helpful, that their very presence becomes helpful by its diversionary – and irritating – nature.

Anyone trying to provide care and support may eventually be able to help the grieving person set limits to their grief, and get them to begin to readjust to 'normal' life – though life may not feel 'normal' to them, possibly ever again. But, whilst people go through all sorts of emotional adjustments in the process of coming to terms with their forthcoming death or bereavement, there are some circumstances where the dying person has particular adjustments to make that are not absolutely run of the mill. That applies especially after an accident, or in certain sorts of illness, where we often have some difficulty in coming to terms with a 'change of body image'. We worry about what will happen to the family left behind, and often want, and even try, to plan for our family and friends 'beyond the grave' to make sure everything goes according to plan, as if somehow our unexpected death can possibly be perceived as fitting into any kind of plan (or even our expected and anticipated death, for, however expected, death always comes as a shock to those left behind).

The family

In all these matters, the exploration of grief and the sharing of it, can bring a family closer together. If things go well, the family experiences the stages of grief together. They are prepared to talk about things that matter. The dying person, if he or she is an adult or a child old enough to have these sorts of conversations, can tell the others what his hopes and fears were and are, and can say something of what he or she would like to see in the future. But there is also something about being with someone we love when they are dying, actually holding their hand. None of us should die alone, and the vision still haunts me of people pushed into a side ward in hospitals in the past and left to get on with the process of dying, alone, seeing their frightened eyes and the loneliness overcoming them before they are even dead. But, where there is an important relationship, then being as near as one can be, holding the person, being with them, experiencing as much of the dying moments as it is possible to share, can be very rewarding. Where there is family or close friends, the more that can be done to encourage them to be there at the time, the better. The more they can be encouraged to sit and hold a hand, or talk lovingly to the person, the better, for many say that the sense of hearing is the last to go. Both the dying person and those who are left are enormously enriched by doing this.

The reason this is so important and I am writing so emphatically about it, is that, when one watches it, seeing people hold the hand of a loved one and talking to them, one realises that they too get a sense of assuaging of the bitterest pangs of grief. They have been there. They have done all they could. It was not frightening. It was, indeed, gentle, and shared. I therefore feel that all that can be done to encourage this, and to make death a gentle process, should be done. This is, with one's loved ones, undoubtedly 'a good death', a 'better way to go'.

There are some who have curious experiences as they approach their own deaths, and others who record near-death experiences when having major (usually open heart or life-support) surgery. In her book *Death and the Family*, Lily Pincus (1976) makes reference to the strange reports of some patients near to the time of death who have come back briefly into consciousness and reported experiencing 'another world'. Many people have doubted such experiences, but too many have reported seeing or feeling this, and therefore it is vital that we do not rubbish such reports, but listen, and ask intelligent questions, and accept this as an experience which was gone though, whether in 'reality', whatever that may mean, or in the imagination, being really irrelevant.

But, the fact that people have these experiences means that, whatever anyone else around thinks, it is important not to interfere, through drugs, thoughtlessness or impatience, with what may well be someone who is dying's most important experience. People's experience of dying can be enormously important to them, and some record what they have felt in vivid prose, very important to those who face their own death. One of my favourite accounts of this kind was *In the Face of Death*, written by Peter Noll, a highly intelligent Swiss man, son of a pastor, whose funeral was conducted by an agnostic. He decided to forego the conventional treatment for his cancer, having read about the effects it could have, and live his life and death.

Peter Noll did not want conventional treatment. He had also watched his father die, and knew that he wanted to keep a record of what happened to him. That account is one of the most moving and beautiful accounts of how small pleasures became important, the value of scenery, the extraordinary reaction to foods and drink and music, whilst some of the important things, the political issues of the day, diminished in importance as he began to realise that things are discussed by human beings as if they were immortal, just as he was all too aware of his own mortality. Many of his readers, near death themselves, have been helped by such stories.

Many of the sentiments experienced by the dying person are shared, in lesser ways perhaps, by those of us they leave behind, and those who have an emotional attachment to them who are also caring for them in those last days, weeks and months. They too sense the loss, the finality of it. They too begin to mourn, but they can also see their lives stretching on beyond the anticipated death, sometimes seeing it with a horror they do not wish the dying loved person to know.

Elderly people dying

For many elderly people this is particularly true. Life has not been easy as they have got older, but they have managed with all the vicissitudes of getting old and less able – together. Then one partner is dying. The other – they are fully dependent the one on the other – wants to care as best as he or she can for the one who is dying, but also faces long years ahead, in a sense frightened of not being able to cope, of being a burden, of being lonely, of losing meaning to life. That grief, that expression of fear, is very real for many elderly people losing a life partner, and should be taken seriously by any of us in any caring role, whether healthcare professional, or pastoral carer such as clergy or counsellor, or family member. The one who is going to survive needs more support, very often, in this kind of situation, than the one who is dying.

This, in its turn, can put a great deal of pressure on children of an elderly couple, these days themselves often getting on in years. If the couple where one is dying are in their eighties, it is not unusual for the children to be in their sixties, and to be facing years of supporting one bereaved parent who feels abandoned, alone and useless, as well as dependent, as they see themselves slipping into dependency as well. These emotions are often all too present around a deathbed of an elderly person, and we need to watch for them, and speak of them. Partly, they need to be watched for because the one who will be left has good reason to fear his or her widowhood – it may well be lonely, and dependent, and we may well feel useless, as society becomes less and less tolerant of the very old.

That is all the more important in the case of people who die in nursing homes, or those who are widowed and living in residential care or nursing homes. Some of these institutions are absolutely excellent in providing support and care to the dying and the bereaved. But others are poor in the extreme, and often regard death as the only way out of the place (all too often, only too true) and some kind of norm, and can unwittingly be quite cruel. In some circumstances, palliative care teams and bereavement services do not go into the nursing homes and care homes, on the basis that the residents are already receiving care. This is a huge mistake, and it is essential that healthcare professionals, social workers, care assistants and families and friends keep a close eye on those who are dying in institutional care, and on those who are bereaved, living in institutions, in order that they get the support and care that is their right, and that others, elsewhere, would expect as the norm.

Dying out of turn – child before parent

But there are other emotions we find around the bedside of a dying person. If the person concerned is younger, is dying 'out of turn', as it were, that brings its own terrible emotions with it. Elderly parents sitting round the deathbed of a terminally ill only daughter, for instance, leaving motherless children and a husband with whom the parents do not get on too well, is one classic case. So is the case of elderly parents sitting by the bed of a much loved son who is also leaving a wife and children, and too little financial provision for them. Or, there are younger parents sitting by the bed of a teenager or young boy or girl in his or her twenties, victims of terrible accidents, or one who contracted an acute, and in this particular case, untreatable, myeloid leukaemia. The list goes on and on. But what is significant is the fact that these 'out of the correct order' deaths have a powerful effect on the family. Most of us can accept, albeit unwillingly, that, as we get older, a spouse will die. As middle-aged children, we know we will lose elderly parents. That is the way of the world. But the death of a child out of order, the death of a sibling out of order, the death of a friend at a young age – somehow that is less acceptable, therefore less absorbable, therefore less tolerable. The reaction is even more agonised, for the pain is not only the pain of loss, but of injustice as well, and the pain of not knowing how to cope is even greater.

Children and grief

Grieving children can often be helped by helping the bereaved parent. But they also need to be allowed to express their grief differently. Adults use words children often do not understand. Their ways of expressing grief are different, and may seem to adults to be uncaring. Often, children need very specialised help in learning to grieve, because the loss of a parent in childhood is no longer a commonplace event. Much of a child's grief may be a reflection of the parent's. If the adult can be encouraged to express feelings, and told firmly that it is beneficial for the child to do likewise, both parent and child can be helped. But they need to recognise that they may mourn in different ways. Small children often draw their loss, whilst adults rarely do, unless they are artists. Children play games that have some macabre purpose – to an adult observer – but are ways of expressing grief. Adults sit and talk, whilst the children get bored. Children will dress up in the dead parent's clothes, whilst adults find it distasteful, almost spooky, to see an eight-year old girl wandering round the house and garden in the mother's high-heeled shoes, two days after her death. But human beings need to mourn in response to loss, and they will do it in different ways at different ages and stages. If they are denied the chance, they suffer in a variety of ways.

It is worth reflecting that human beings are animals, and watching animals grieve is often helpful. When our cat lost her twin brother in a road accident, she moped for weeks. She was looking for him to play with, and, indeed, since he was always the bold one, to take her on journeys and to protect her from attackers. (She was the most unadventurous and wimpish of cats. Any bird she ever managed to catch to bring us as an unwelcome offering had to be so old and incapacitated as to be better caught by her than by some nastier, more vicious creature.) Dogs mope too when they lose a sibling, and especially an owner. The story of 'Greyfriars' Bobby', the dog that sat by his master's grave for a decade or more in Edinburgh, is a case in point. If we can see it in animals, why should we wish to deny it to any human beings? And yet we do. Until very recently, it was felt better for children not to express their grief, and particularly not to be present at the funeral – as if somehow, if they had no closure in a ceremony, their pain would be less great. The damage done to them psychologically by that view (presumably with its roots in the upset that parents and other adults felt at children expressing their grief) must have been enormous, even incalculable.

Siblings

Children, however painful it is, must be told about the possible death of a sibling, or of a parent. To simply say, after a sister has died, that she has gone away and is not coming back, is cruel beyond belief – the child who is left behind will imagine the most dreadful things and may well think that the brother or sister going away was his or her fault. Children, just like adults, need to be prepared for an expected death, and, when death comes unexpectedly, they need to have it explained to them, and to be allowed to share in the grieving process, and the rituals.

It used to be common not to take children to the funerals of family members, because 'it would be too upsetting'. Clearly, it was not that 'it was too upsetting' for the children, but actually for the adults who had to take them, and who would then have to watch the children's grief and think of them as motherless waifs or as vulnerable accident-prone beings. But children need to be included. They mourn and grieve. They may not express it as adults do, but that is no excuse for excluding them from the process, for they have much to gain, in terms of their own later development, from having been included from the very earliest stage.

The death of babies

One special category here is the death of babies, and even still-born children. Modern children quite rightly understand about pregnancy. They often touch their mother's stomachs and feel the baby kicking. Should the baby die at a very tender age of a few hours or days, or even be still-born at the end, it is vitally important that the older children should be included in grieving for this loss of new life. It is even more important when one considers that it used to be the case, particularly in Judaism and Islam (and to some extent still is), that a baby under 30 days old was not given a full funeral. The mourning process was curtailed, and the baby often buried in an unmarked grave. In my view, that was a system invented by men, who did not under-stand the powerful emotions of giving birth to a new life, however short-lived. There are those who argue it was merely practical, because infant death was so common. But the fact something is common does not make it less sad. The loss is the same whether it has happened before or not, until we become so numb from repeated pain we can grieve no longer. Most of us will never be in that position, and therefore grieving for a tiny baby or still-born child is important to us, and to the other children in the family. They need to know what has happened. Ideally, they should see the child, and touch it, so that its death holds no terrors for them. Certainly, some form of ritual should be held for a small baby as well, and other children included in it, so that they will understand, and experience death as desperately sad, but not necessarily frightening.

Healthcare professionals working in the field of neonatal care and in mater-nity units, need to understand about this. Many are very good at encouraging the families to mourn this tiny being, but some still have not realised that, in these days of rare infant mortality, other children will fear that they too are going to die, and need to have it explained to them very carefully. Often, healthcare professionals are the best at doing this, because they can explain to the children what it was that was wrong with the baby that made it die. That in itself is reassuring, since it means that they can understand that there was an illness or something wrong, rather than it just being an accident.

Still-births

But the effect of a still-birth is even more complicated. Until recently, still-born babies were simply taken away and never seen by the mothers, let alone the rest of the family. It was as though nine months of pregnancy had never been. Yet the mothers and their other children, and the fathers, and the rest of the family, had often lived along with that pregnancy and lived with the expectation of the baby. The modern trend to take the death of a still-born child seriously is much to be welcomed, but it also needs to be watched care-fully. It should not be sentimentalised. It should be treated as an awful thing to have happened, ideally with some kind of medical explanation as to why it did. The tendency to take photographs of the still-born child, as if it had lived, is one we should encourage, for it allows the grieving family to focus on a real being whom they can envisage, even though they never got the chance to know the still-born child as a person.

These are some examples of the variation in the ways people will grieve, adults and children, for parents, spouses, children and friends – and for still-born babies who never really lived. There are countless other categories and examples, too many to go through. But it is important for those who are bereaved themselves, and those who work with them to realise that grief comes in many ways, is demonstrated in many ways, and that, however difficult it is to recognise its symptoms, we must realise that when we are grieving, we will behave differently, unable to help it, and that we will be beset by physical signs of grief that are completely unexpected, about which nobody ever tells you – such as extreme exhaustion. When my father died, I could not believe how tired I was, having done little physical work or intel-lectual activity for days. Indeed, I would go to bed early, and wake up late, and be more exhausted in the morning than I had been the night before. This is not abnormal. It is a common phenomenon amongst those who are grief-stricken – but nobody thinks to tell you. Similarly, though people tell you that your appetite for food and drink may be much reduced, and though those who come to comfort you may produce food to tempt you, to make sure you eat, no-one tells you in advance that your tastes may actually change for the duration, or that some particular foods may become revolting to you, for no apparent reason. Yet others who have been through the grieving process say that they too have had similar experiences. All one can say is that grief strikes us in different ways, but that it is a form of journey, a process we have to go through, and somehow pull ourselves out the other side, with a little help from our friends and various professionals who are there to support us, with all the odd phenomena that happen in the midst of it. Those of us who are grief-stricken need to know that is likely, as do those who care for us, professionally or as family and friends; we need to under-stand that grief is the way the human body and mind eventually work through appalling loss, and that we need to experience it, however horrible, without antidepressants, without being made the objects of study as if somehow we were abnormal, over-reacting, lacking self-control. For grief hurts. It is painful. But it is painful because it is our way of processing the most painful events imaginable – the loss of our nearest and dearest. And we must be allowed to mourn, to grieve, to come to terms, to accept loss, and to carry on living with the best of memories, and the sense that we experienced the loss fully and well.

So, we need to learn a new vocabulary. Some of it can be learned from the textbooks on grieving, from Colin Murray Parkes, from Elisabeth Kubler-Ross, from Dora Black, from Lily Pincus. But some of it cannot be learned from the 'experts'. Some of it will have to come from exploring emotions each of us holds as individuals. We have to think about what we feel about dying – our own deaths, the deaths of loved ones, and then use that personal thinking to inform our relationship with those we care for. That does not mean for one single minute that we should inflict our views on our patients. Far from it. But without thinking about what death means to us as indivi-duals, we are unlikely to be able to help those who are facing their own deaths, or the deaths of loved ones, come to terms with what they can see dimly, through acute misery. Our own thinking, our own desire to work out our own reactions, will help us support others in their grief, and is, therefore, critically important for us to do.

3

The role of helpers

Introduction

Professional: general

Healthcare staff have a crucial role when someone is dying. They are there, watching. They know what the likely course of events will be. They may well have provided much of the interventionist care in the first place. They will continue to provide some forms of care, and some of them will provide comfort. Some healthcare professionals find caring for the dying immensely rewarding, and do a great deal of the pastoral care themselves, usually within a team of palliative care professionals and district nurses, working alongside hospital consultants of various kinds and general practitioners (GPs). Some healthcare professionals find the whole area of terminal care too difficult. They feel that they have done their job when it gets to the point that there is nothing more to be done in the interventionist sense. They will often hand over to the GPs, if the dying person is at home, or to the palliative care specialists in hospitals.

But, in many cases, the ideal team is not present for all sorts of reasons, and other people who end up caring for someone who is dying will be a mixture of those with specialist training, and a considerable interest in the work, and those for whom it is a relatively small part of their general role, such as some GPs and some district nurses.

But, whatever the situation, any team of people looking after someone who is dying and his or her family can bring in other professionals, such as counsellors and pastors. They can and should do so if that is what the family wants. But many families do not want any such thing. And the healthcare professionals find themselves in the situation of being dispassionate obser-vers, watching a family, or a group or a couple in pain. Sometimes, by simply stopping and listening and talking, they can help. The odd word that acknowledges how difficult and painful the situation is may well be very helpful. Precisely those families who do not want the counsellor or the priest will often take a word of comfort, a word of acknowledgement of pain, from a healthcare professional. For the doctor or nurse is not someone who will necessarily invade their space, as they perceive a counsellor or priest might. The doctor or nurse is a professional, there to look after one's bodily needs when things go wrong, as in this case they undoubtedly have. It is, therefore, quite appropriate for the doctor or nurse to notice the pain, and comment on it. And it can be very helpful.

But all this presupposes that the person who is dying has been told that that is the case. It is, however, still surprisingly common to find people who are terminally ill who have not actually been told. This does not necessarily mean that they do not know, but it does mean that there has been some kind of unholy alliance between the healthcare professionals and the spouse or other family members who have colluded to agree that 'it would be better' if Dad, or Aunt Jane, or Cissie, or cousin Ali, were not told. This is not always wrong. But it is wrong if the person concerned, who is actually dying, gives an indication that he or she wants honesty in the situation. It is still common to find a situation in a hospital (less common in hospice for obvious reasons, since most people know what hospices are for, and for whom) where the dying person knows he or she is dying, the family knows the person is terminally ill, but each pretends the other does not know. The failure in communication, the lack of grabbing of an opportunity to talk in that situation, is really worrying. Many families never do talk about the things that matter in the normal course of life, but there is something unut-terably sad about a family that continues a defence, and indeed a pretence, to the last, often on the basis they are protecting each other by so doing, and never say the things that matter to each other at all. When the person dies, it is too late, and all the pain and anger and guilt come out, and cannot be resolved as they could have been had the family talked while the now dead person was still alive.

So, though it should never be forced, healthcare professionals, family members, anyone who is around who sees that situation developing, should keep an eye on it, and try as hard as they can to encourage the family to talk. Suggesting is one thing, however. Force, forcing the situation by telling each party that the other knows in their presence, is another, and should never be used. Some families, some relationships, have always been fragile, and it is not always possible or desirable to mend the relationship and make it a strong and honest one at a deathbed scene, however satisfactory, in some ways, that might be in a story-book sort of way.

Truth-telling

But, for many health- and social care professionals, that means acquiring a different mind set. It means thinking more and more about how they would feel themselves in the same situation. It also means thinking about the balance between a family's desires and interests, and the dying individual's. For families all too often say that healthcare professionals should do everything possible for someone, even when that individual may not have wished, at a time when they could make their desires clear, to have everything done for them at all. Similarly, dying patients often try to protect their families, and do not tell them what they know. It is quite common to encounter families where the wife will not tell the husband that he is dying, the husband will not talk to the wife about the fact that he knows that he is dying, and they carry on in a misguided attempt to protect each other. The healthcare professionals, in this case very often the nurses, are often the only ones who know that both sides know, husband and wife, what the true prognosis is. They are, then, in the difficult position of deciding whether to tell each partner that the other knows, or whether to leave things as they are, in the assumption that the couple are in some ill-defined way happier like that. He or she would not have wanted to know, and certainly would not have wanted to discuss it.

This is a major difficulty for health- and social care professionals, for it is very likely to be the case that a couple has not discussed issues of their own mortality at all, given the lack of willingness to discuss death at all, more generally, in our society. It is, therefore, possibly true that each is right when they say the other would not have wanted to know or to discuss these things. Yet it can be very difficult for healthcare professionals to work in an environment when it is clear that both parties, and indeed a whole family, know that one of them is dying, but will not discuss it openly. It can make the task of the healthcare professional almost impossible, because he or she is walking through a miry trap of dishonesty and has to watch every word extremely carefully.

Public debate on these issues needs to be encouraged, and public standards established. That applies to the telling of the truth to individuals, as well as to the discussion about how much intensive intervention it is worth trying to do for people who are seriously ill, and arguably dying. That is one of the reasons why values clarification is so important within medical and other healthcare training, and in the wider public debate. The debate about life values needs to be carried out between healthcare professionals and the public in partnership, which is why medical students need so desperately to be pushed into thinking about these issues, and dragged away from the old-fashioned, exhausting, imitative and sometimes destructive apprenticeship model which inhibits thinking about social issues in healthcare. Attitudes to truth, suffering, pain and life expectancy need to be worked out first, and students need to think about whether everything can be done for everybody, or should be. Should we even aim to cure some people? Or should we just care for them, very well?

Costs of caring for the very ill can only be contained in this area if the general view is that it is morally right to do so, and that requires a general debate and a willingness to change on the part of the medical profession which is, as yet, unclear. More importantly, it would make explicit what values about life, health and caring for those who suffer are common within a society. The elderly and terminally ill must not feel they are being denied care they want. But that care might be different from what they get at present, and could mean more palliative care, relieving pain and suffering, more holistic and less scientifically driven, than what is at present available. Indeed, it might be care, rather than attempted, often futile, cure, going higher up the agenda.

How healthcare professionals might help to counsel us

If our aim is to alleviate suffering – by providing care – then we have to go further and ask whether that is only pain, suffering, as perceived by patients and their carers, or whether it is the much broader suffering of an emotional and psychological nature. Is the suffering of an 87-year-old woman who says: 'Leave me alone, I want to die', to be taken seriously by healthcare professionals, or is this a matter for social services and friends and family? Can we do more to help people face their own mortality, and do it within a healthcare setting where people are more likely to accept it than if they have to get special counselling from social workers or counsellors, which they all too frequently resist?

Because in our society people expect to die in a healthcare setting, it may be best to train healthcare professionals to a much higher level than we used to in the field of caring for the terminally ill. Indeed, it could be argued that it should be a part of basic training, something that is only just coming about, and even then with a very short time spent considering terminal care and hospices. The hospice movement itself has done valiantly in the field of training of healthcare professionals, but it has trained those who were already interested. It has not yet become established as a matter of course that all healthcare professionals in their training will do some work on caring for the dying. And it is critical that they do, because they will have to do much of the unofficial counselling, whatever happens. And they need to be able to recognise, not only the fear and the pain, but also the grief on the part of those who are dying, grief at what they are leaving behind, at whom they are leaving behind, at the unfinished business, at the unsorted messes. That grief, that sorrow, that anger has to be recognised and legitimised. Dying people need to know from the people who are looking after them that it is all right to say that they do not wish to go on any more, or that they have no intention of dying right now. Both depression and anger must be recognised. Those feelings must be recognised as common. The comfort of a nurse telling a dying person that what she is feeling is not unusual, when the patient is looking out on a bleak world, without the apparent capacity to do anything but feel tired, in pain, constipated maybe, and miserable, is very considerable. Good nursing, recognising the sorrow and the grief, is of enormous benefit. Yet, quite often, the dying patient has no real language to express that grief. One of the problems of not talking about death and dying for so many decades is that we have lost the language in which to do it. Though we will talk easily of grief, we do not necessarily know what it means, and we do not have the techniques, in conversation, to tease out some of the emotions that make up 'grief', as we term that series of emotions that forms the roller coaster of anticipated or indeed already occurring bereavement.

For many healthcare professionals, this seems almost intolerable, and they rightly ask whether their interests should not be taken into account too. That is an entirely legitimate question. For though one can argue very properly from an ethical standpoint that the paramount interests must be those of the patient him- or herself, that does not apply to the whole family. The interests of the healthcare professionals also have a role here, and they should not be forced to work in an atmosphere of dishonesty, unless they regard it as necessary.

But, increasingly, people are told that they are terminally ill. They are told by their doctors, usually, although sometimes inadvertently by a nurse, who knows the diagnosis and prognosis. Nurses can and should play an important role here. Particularly in a hospital situation, which is often where the first 'telling' takes place, the doctors are lamentably short of time (so are the nurses, in fact) and often do not have the time or skill to tell people well. Though much has been done to improve that situation, especially in the field of communications skills for healthcare professionals in general, including telling bad news, until such a time as all healthcare professionals are trained and skilled in giving bad news, it will continue to be the nurses who are often better than doctors at this particular piece of telling the truth. It is also often the cleaning staff, who are not supposed to be involved at all, who give the most comfort, and tell patients more of what they want to know by their experience of having seen it all before.

However, someone, usually a doctor, tells an individual who is already ill and in hospital that the condition they have is terminal. 'You are not going to get better. We will do all we can to keep you comfortable. I cannot tell you how long it will be.' Terrible words, often baldly spoken. The patient hears this, and will react in many different ways. One of the most common is denial. 'It is not true. It cannot be me. I want a second opinion.' But, after denial, there often comes anger and acceptance. Often, particularly if not elderly already, the person is terribly angry, taking it out on the person who tells him or her, on the nursing staff, on his or her family, the nearest and dearest, who can have a rough time with it. Nor is it always easy to do the telling, however well-trained one has been. For one's own emotions come into play. To see the pain spread across someone's face, to see the tears form, is never easy even for hardened health professionals who have to do it all the time (one of the reasons some become hardened). Indeed, there are always problems because many patients will say that they want only to be told the truth, but when they are given the truth as they have requested, it becomes clear that they did not want to know. They wish they had not been told, yet it is very difficult to plan future care without telling the truth to someone who has always demanded it, someone who has been apparently emotionally tough and resilient all his or her life.

The health professional's response

Professional: general

Thinking in terms of what the individual might prefer, and what the individual's values and preferences might be, is hard for any health professional. Health professionals in general, and doctors in particular, have traditionally been educated in a particular way. They have largely been exposed to an apprenticeship model of training, where the best student is the one who best emulates the senior person on whose 'firm' he or she is. Though training has changed dramatically in recent years, and ethics and values play a greater part in early training, there still tends to be little discussion of values once on the ward, of what makes treatment right or wrong, of what the relationship between patient and doctor should be. And advance directives, discussed below, are still relatively rare, so that being clear about a patient's preferences – if the patient cannot or does not say him or herself – is still far from easy. If the senior healthcare professionals do not make a huge effort themselves to find out what the patient wants – though increasingly they do – then younger doctors and nurses in training will still make an assumption that they are being given an example of good practice by their seniors, which they would do well to emulate.

Nor is there much discussion about cultural and religious differences, both in ritual matters, but also in values terms, which is very important for health professionals dealing with patients, caring for people, whose cultural, and religious background is different from their own. It is undoubtedly useful to understand something about the culture and faith to which the person they are looking after belongs, or to which they are actively seeking a final return. It is particularly important where the family is profoundly involved in the religion or culture concerned, where it is possible to cause great offence by doing the wrong thing. For that reason, over the last 25 years or so, I have been writing and lecturing on the subject of caring for dying people of different faiths and cultures, simply because there is a great deal to be gained for all concerned from getting it right. We cannot be expected to get it completely right either, but the fact that we have tried, the fact that we are prepared to ask questions of the individual and the family to make sure we are doing the right thing, gives a strong sense of reassurance to the people concerned.

The worst form of paternalism in healthcare is not the intervention which is done because the healthcare professional thinks it the best thing to do in the circumstances – after all, that is done relying very properly on the professional judgement of the professional. The worst thing is where the religious and cultural attitudes of the caring professional are in some paternalistic way – often for the best of motives – inflicted on a patient who holds very different views, beliefs and attitudes.

I speak as someone who has experienced this. A profoundly believing Christian nurse, when I was seriously ill in my mid-twenties, tried to comfort me with hope in the hereafter 'in the arms of Jesus'. As a believing Jewess, and as someone then training to be a rabbi, I found this curiously offensive, and felt I wanted my faith left alone, that it was an improper use of the intimacy engendered by being dependent when seriously ill. She had meant well, but unwittingly she caused considerable upset and offence. It is something which can easily be avoided with a bit of knowledge, a great deal of care, and a willingness to ask questions of the people for whom one is caring and their family and friends. Most people are delighted that caring professional staff are showing an interest and actually want to know.

The healthcare professionals who were close to the person who has died have a clear role to play in both helping to give the religious leader who is going to conduct a funeral information about the person who has died, if he or she did not know him or her well, and in going to the funeral. It is amazing how comforting the family of someone who has died often find it if those who have looked after their nearest and dearest in the weeks and months before the death actually come to the funeral. There is something about the very intimacy of the care that was given which makes the act of going to the funeral very welcome, and somehow sets the seal of the relationship the healthcare professional had with the person who is now dead, and whose life is being remembered.

Things are changing in that direction. Many National Health Service (NHS) employers actively encourage staff, particularly in the community, to attend the funeral of someone they have cared for long term, and encourage them, too, to continue to support the family longer term, even though that is not normally seen as part of the role of the district nurse or the GP. But that role is changing, and a sense of being part of a wider community is pervading primary care, allowing this kind of reaching out to take place on a more regular and frequent basis.

For some of these issues have been being addressed in the teaching of young medical and other health- and social care professional students for the last 20 years or so, and changes are beginning to be rooted into the culture.

Indeed, there are textbooks which try to think through the relationship between professional and patient, in a way quite different from the old-fashioned, well-established, straight apprenticeship model. Downie and Calman, in their excellent and pioneering volume, *Healthy Respect* (1987), suggested that:

> *The following list gives an idea of the wide variety of roles that any healthcare professional might adopt:*
>
> *Healer: The primary function here is one of caring and healing. All professional healthcare groups have this as a basic function.*
> *Technician: There is a technical role in almost all professional activities, whether it is in performing an operation, dressing a wound, massaging a leg, pulling a tooth, or knowing the relevant section of welfare legislation.*
> *Counsellor: Much of the routine work of healthcare workers is dealing with the psychological and social problems of patients and their families. In some instances, this may even overlap with the spiritual area.*
> *Educator: Teaching is an important role of those who work in the health service. This may involve professional, public or patient education.*
> *Scientist: Most groups have a responsibility to develop new ideas and to investigate the causes and treatment of disease.*
> *Friend: In some areas of clinical practice it is not difficult to become friends with the patient and the family. In some instances this may mean that the professional role, for example, as a healer, may conflict with the role as a friend.*
> *Political: Doctors, nurses and other healthcare workers, because of their special knowledge, may, because they feel strongly about it, become involved in political activities. Campaigns against cigarette smoking, drugs or alcohol abuse, or nuclear power, are obvious areas of involvement.*

These are some aspects of the role of the professional healthcare worker. They are confused roles in many cases, with conflicting values. The conflict between the role of friend and healer can be considerable, as can the conflict between the role of genuine scientist and friend, that between the politician and friend, or the politician and healer, or indeed that between the technician and friend. For instance, no friend likes to hurt a friend, even for the best of reasons. It is, therefore, often hard for doctors who are close friends of their patients to perform such relatively simple things as minor surgical procedures, or, more alarming to many, to prescribe drugs of which the side-effects themselves are known to be unpleasant. The doctor can say to him- or herself that he or she knows perfectly well that it is in the patient's friend's interest for him or her to do so, and it can be done with consent and, indeed, with the fullest of information, wholly respecting the patient's friend's autonomy. But it does not make it any easier, in exactly the same way as it is never easy for doctors to treat their own families.

The same conflict occurs over the scientific process. A good scientist has a real curiosity about conditions and causes. Scientific values are about finding out truths, investigating, experimenting in order to further human knowledge. A doctor, whether in general practice or in hospital medicine, may well be conducting some form of research, satisfying that natural curiosity which may be one element of what involved him or her in medicine in the first place. But it is remarkably difficult to include a friend in any randomised controlled trial. The whole point of such a trial is that neither the patient nor the doctor should know which arm of the trial the patient is in, so that for a friend to put a friend into such a blind study goes against the comforting and supportive values of friendship, and can be extraordinarily difficult. All the theorising in the world about how it may be therapeutic, because the patient may end up in the arm of the trial that has the most beneficial treatment, does not help in explaining to a friend that no-one knows the best treatment, and that a trial is taking place, and it might be good and it might not, and little is known about the side-effects (or there would not be a trial) and that really there is not much comfort one can give.

These are real conflicts. Indeed, one might argue that it is extremely difficult to act professionally, as a doctor should, with a patient who is also a close friend. The desire with a friend is to give comfort, to be supportive, to be kind. But in treatment it may be necessary to be cruel to be kind, and the coping with uncertainty with a friend or family member is often worse than it is with someone more distant, hard though it is at any time. All this is difficult whenever any conflict occurs, but it is very much more difficult when it is a case of terminal illness, when the decisions which are made are likely to be the last significant ones about healthcare for the person concerned.

These are the kinds of issues young healthcare professionals have to think about. They have to think beyond the four principles of medical ethics which are normally cited – of beneficence, of non-maleficence, of justice and of respect for autonomy – and look at what it is that is expected of them and how these roles, and their underlying values, might conflict. And those conflicts are even worse when the person is terminally ill, or probably so, and even worse when the healthcare professional knows that a trial is taking place which is of enormous scientific significance – but not to the person in front of them, who is dying anyway. And across the health professional's mind drifts the awful thought of whether it is morally acceptable to ask a dying person to be altruistic.

Is it? The examples are always given of terrible air crashes where cannibalism is the only hope of survival, and the oldest and illest say, altruistically, 'Eat me'. But this is rather different. This is an extreme situation for the patient, but not for everyone else who is treating him or her. Can someone who is so ill really be asked to go through a clinical trial of a drug, unpleasant in its side-effects, for the benefit of a future he or she will never know?

The doctor's role

And the friend/scientist or friend/healer conflicts are only two of many possible ones, such as the obvious conflict between trying to do the best for the individual patient, there before you at that time, and looking at resources available for the totality of patients, when there is never enough to provide everything possible for all. So the drug that may give someone a longer life but has appalling side-effects, such as extreme nausea, can only be counteracted by the giving of large doses of a very expensive anti-emetic. Should the person who is probably dying be given such expensive drugs, since the chances are not high anyway? Or should the expensive drugs be kept for those more likely to survive? And is giving an anti-emetic really important compared with giving the chemotherapeutic drug which may actually extend life? These are real decisions to be made by health professionals. But they impact heavily on patient care. And the terminally ill patient may have different answers, seeing things from a different perspective, from the one the health professionals would normally come to for the quality of a very small amount of life remaining becomes enormously important.

For the doctor is likely to think: Which do you have in mind with this patient before you? The individual? Or the sense of the public good, the totality of the patient population? Do you spend your budget on treatment with a poor success rate, but something, right now, for this patient who has a poor prognosis, and is probably dying anyway, or save the money for the next patient, who may or may not come with a condition where the treatment is expensive, but more successful? And, in all this, do you tell the patients the truth, about what treatments cost, about the likely outcomes, and about how you make your decisions? And are you, as a health professional, genuinely acting in the individual patient's interest, if you do not discuss it? Or, is the doctor merely using his or her value system to decide for each individual patient?

Doctors have not, on the whole, wanted to take this complex series of questions on board. The UK Patient's Charter made it clear from the early 1990s that doctors had to ask for consent to treatment. Professional guidelines and standards had asked for proper consent to be sought and given long before that, but how that consent was sought has always been a matter of debate. Equally, with people who are dying, there are questions about whether they have written an advance directive (living will) or not, and whether they have made a clear decision on what they want to happen if they are not capable of saying at the time. Or, have they appointed a healthcare proxy, someone who has formally been given the role of making decisions if they are not capable of making them themselves? These are relatively new questions for healthcare professionals, which cut across the old ones about resources and whether something is 'worth' doing. But, the change of emphasis from the patient being someone who did what he or she was told, in a relatively paternalistic model, to one where the patient (the person who is dying makes his or her own decisions within the framework of what is available, has changed the dynamic of relationships very considerably. So when consent is sought, it may not necessarily include details of cost and resource allocation, of public concern versus the individual concern for the patient facing you right now. Yet patients should be told something of the risks, something of what the treatment will really be like. And when someone is dying, with only a short time ahead of them, then that need to know becomes all the more acute. Yet, often, they are not told, and, if they were, health professionals know that patients would often make other decisions, as the doctors themselves would. Hence the increasing need for advance directives, and clear instructions about what all of us would like to happen in those end-of-life situations.

There is a fear amongst the medical professionals and amongst patient groups that we might go down the US road, with doctors held in scant respect, being seen as driven wholly by the prospect of financial gain, merely out for a quick buck, and with little in the way of real professional values. That does not need to be so. Doctors have lost some public respect in recent years in this country. They are no longer quite as popular in the public mind as they once were. They do not have the reputation nurses have for tenderness and for being on the side of the patient, though it is questionable whether nurses are always as much on the side of the patient, the patient's advocate, as they sometimes claim to be, since they, too, have professional interests that may not be those of the patients, and their very mode of organisation, in hierarchical, task-oriented structures on the whole, is inimical to making close relationships with the patients in their care. But doctors are still felt to be good people, with the patients' interests at heart, and able to make sensible decisions, in the patients' interest.

It is these issues, these questions about allocation of resources, the fact that it will be wholly obvious, in the widest of possible public arenas, that doctors are having to give thought to the relative costs of treatments and procedures, and for whom they are intended (old, young, dying, likely to survive), that so terrifies doctors themselves. They do not want to have to say to patients that a particular treatment is too expensive. They do not want to have to say to someone who is dying that there is some treatment they cannot have that would alleviate their symptoms, even if it cannot possibly cure them. Nor do they want to talk about the financial implications of all sorts of other areas of practice, such as the fact that for most, but not all, clinical trials, particularly those sponsored by the pharmaceutical companies, doctors are paid for entering patients in a trial. To add to this, they are paid on a per capita basis, according to the numbers they recruit into the trial, a practice which is still more or less universal despite the Royal College of Physicians coming out strongly against it and arguing that it is unethical (RCP, 1990). And whilst in hospital practice these monies tend to go into research funds for the department concerned, in the case of general practice, this money goes to the individual GP or the practice. Yet how many patients know this when they consent to enter a trial? And dying patients may feel they have a duty to help future generations. And on what basis, if respecting the patients' interests is a key professional value, is it legitimate to keep the financial implications of a trial from him or her? And how can we justify this to terminally ill patients? Yet the side-effects could be argued to matter less to the dying.

Very few young healthcare professionals in training or recently out of medical school could even begin to go through these discussions. Despite the insistence on the four principles of medical ethics as cited in Beauchamp and Childress (1989), the majority of medical students still cover relatively limited discussions on medical ethics in their training even now. Their ability to argue through these puzzles, and work out for themselves their beliefs about what is right and wrong, tends to be decidedly weak. And that must be disturbing for patients, who want to know what the professionals think as well as what they think themselves, so they can make up their own minds about what to do.

Doctors must know what it is they believe in and be able to convey that both to their patients and to the public. Patients who are dying, or who are seriously ill and believe that they may be dying, need to be able to talk properly to their healthcare professional advisors. Doctors can no longer stand by and say that the only really unethical behaviour is sexual misconduct with a patient. (It has been an enormous improvement to see poor performance *per se* given as a reason for disciplinary action by the General Medical Council since the early 1990s, and put into effect in the early years of this millennium, for it is on the good performance, and fine care, of doctors, that the public relies.) It is, arguably, unethical to give a patient advice that is not in his or her best interests. It is certainly unethical to do it for personal benefit, and it is vital to consider the value system of the patient as much as, if not more than, one's own. And when it comes to the dying patient, that imperative has to be written very large. And, if one does not know the values of the patient, and that person is no longer able to discuss such matters, though the health professional should have tried to have the discussion earlier where possible, then the doctors and nurses should ask the family, the members of the family who are soon to be bereaved – and it is not easy. This is one strong argument – even if we accepted no other – for encouraging all of us to write advance directives or appoint a formal healthcare proxy.

Indeed, it is an object lesson for health professionals to read accounts of how individuals make decisions for themselves. To read the intelligent reaction of someone who knows something about what the treatment might be for a particular condition and decides to forego it on the basis that he or she would rather be aware, would rather not be, in Peter Noll's words as quoted by Max Frisch at his funeral, 'a disabled object of medicine'. There are many amongst us who regard the treatment of some conditions as worse than the disease.

There are many who say that if they had known what the chemotherapy would be like, they would not have had it. And there are those who, if they had understood the likelihood of the treatment effecting no cure, but only, if that, a short increase in the number of days, weeks or months, yet not necessarily in their quality, would have said no. Health professionals bear a huge responsibility here. If they are facing someone with a truly serious, life-threatening condition, they must not use their values, or indeed their scientific curiosity, as a means of making the decision. Indeed, it is arguable whether they should make the decision at all.

The first role for doctors in this situation is therefore to find out, as best they can, what the individual patient wants or would have wanted if he or she could express him or herself. The second duty must be to act on that information, and to regard it as a professional imperative to treat someone as they wished to be treated, right to the end, except where the desire of the individual patient is against the law, as in the case of euthanasia, for instance, or simply impracticable, such as to go home when there is no-one at home to provide the care.

The second main role of the doctor, when it comes to the final stage of someone's dying and they are in charge, as GP or as consultant, is to do everything to alleviate pain where that is wished for. For that, the work has to be done as a team. Doctors, nurses, specialist palliative care nurses, the hospice movement, all need to work together. The best experiences, the best deaths, the most satisfying for the individuals and those around them, seem to be when the team get it absolutely right. And that means building up a considerable level of trust between professionals in a short space of time.

It also does not necessarily mean the doctor being the team leader, for very often it is the nurses who provide the majority of the care, and who know what the patient wants and needs better than the doctor. One of the great skills of a doctor is to know just how much to trust the team, and when to leave the team to make the decisions themselves, without the doctor, who comes in and out, interfering beyond prescribing and asking questions and giving advice.

For instance, in the case of my father's death, the nurses largely took charge. He was cared for in hospital until some 30 hours before his death. He desperately wanted to go home, so it was set up for him to do so, though it took a little time to arrange, particularly as it was over a Bank Holiday, always a problematic time for services. In hospital, his care was provided by superb nurses who were primarily coronary care nurses, but of whom several had an interest in terminal care. He was kept comfortable, encouraged to go out during the day, counselled by one of the nurses in particular, given tender loving care, all under the guidance of a particular consultant whose ward had a very high level of nursing skill and a considerable team spirit.

When he came home, care was transferred to the GP, who was away, and it was therefore his locum who took charge, alongside the district nurses, who were wonderful and could not have done more for us. There were also specialist palliative care nurses who kept an eye on what was going on, and soon there were Marie Curie nurses with him all the time, to keep him comfortable, because he became too ill for us to manage.

The team, once we were at home, did not all know each other. Yet, they built up a level of professional trust and care between them remarkably quickly. Their skill in passing information one to another was one of the things that made my father's death such a good one. For they got the feeling about how quickly things were going, and encouraged my father to do what he could while he could, and then encouraged us to sit with him, holding his hand and talking to him, whilst ensuring that he did not become agitated, but remained peaceful.

And it was a very peaceful end, as he wanted it, at home, provided for him by people who were working together, at least in part, for the first time, and whose desire was to get it right for my father, the person who was their prime focus of care, and us. Seeing the team get it right was something quite remarkable. The GP made the bed up with the district nurse whilst I held my father. The night district nurse spent time comforting me, whilst her colleague helped the Marie Curie nurse turn my father. And so on, and so on. It is much harder to get that kind of team care working in people's homes, yet it is probably where it is most important, because most people, given the choice, would prefer to die at home.

To some extent, that has been helped by hospice homecare teams, working with district nurses and GPs. They can give some of their expertise to a team that regularly works over a particular patch, where the district nurses work regularly with a particular GP anyway, and therefore skilled hospice outreach teams can help build up a regular team for providing the best kind of pallia- tive care at home. But it does not always work, and it is in the nature of the teams that the quality of care rests.

Nurses' role

Nurses, more than many other health professionals, are well used to working in teams, particularly in the community. And nursing is a profession well- adjusted to working in people's homes. Nurses who work in the community have seen everything, more or less, and know how people live, in what squalor, or with what idiosyncrasies, or in what splendour. Nurses in the community are more aware of cultural and religious variations in families, because they see them at home. Nurses are also trained to be natural negotia- tors, because of the way they have to work with each other and with doctors. Once they are taken away from the hierarchical structure of nursing in a ward in hospital, they actually find themselves in a situation where much of their practice depends on great negotiation skills. Certainly in the terminal care field that is a vital talent to have; being able to negotiate with families, and with individuals, being able to persuade various service providers to bring supplies, being able to get drugs, special mattresses, backrests and so on, just when you need them, is no mean feat. District nurses build up phenomenally good relationships with those who provide home loans, both in the health services and from local authorities. They learn to work the system, whatever it might be locally, and they are able to get things done that private individuals take weeks to achieve.

That is a much underrated skill that district nurses, in particular, have. Yet, in order to provide good terminal care at home, having the right supplies of drugs and supplies of all sorts of disposable equipment and aids, is essential.

So nurses do not only provide practical care, physically. They also take charge of getting all the things needed to make a dying person comfortable, and they take a load off the family, who cannot cope at that time with many of the practical demands, when they need to get hold of things they have never needed before.

But nurses do much more than that. Indeed, nurses, and doctors, at home, provide a great deal of the unofficial counselling, help, support and advice, both for the individual patient and for the family or friends caring for him or her. And they regularly do it extremely well, though in many cases they are helped by being given specific training, either in terminal care, or sometimes in counselling.

But they have an important role to play in terminal care. For instance, healthcare staff need to make sure that those who have no-one to care for them, no family and few friends, do not die alone. People should not die isolated, lonely and frightened, any more than they should be left, as they often are, in the corridor of a hospital, waiting for some frightening procedure to be done to them, such as an angiogram, when they are wide awake – alone. None of us should be left alone like that. It is unkind, and it is certainly not acceptable under the generic label of 'healthcare'. For care requires emotional awareness, all too often missing.

Yet nurses are often able to deal with this kind of situation. First, if they are community nurses, they often know who has no-one, either from the person him- or herself or from his or her neighbours and others locally. It is one of the great advantages in Britain of having a primary care system with general practice and district nurses, as it allows health professionals to know a considerable amount about the social circumstances of many of the people with whom health services come into contact.

Nurses often deal with those who have no-one, and provide the care, comfort and spiritual care (in some cases) they crave as they are dying. Often it seems that nurses go back to the Nightingale image of the 'lady with the lamp' when they provide care to those who have no-one at the end of their lives. They do, literally, bring hope and comfort to many, and should be encouraged to do so.

So one of the main roles of nurses in terminal care is to pick up the needs of those who are dying, to be key members of teams, taking advice where it is offered, working closely with other professionals, but also using their community knowledge, in many cases, to find out what is needed, and to provide it.

Nurses are key players in terminal care. Though many patients need drugs, particularly careful doses, and careful titration of doses of pain controlling drugs such a morphine, which is prescribed by doctors, it is nurses who get the dosage right, and who watch for signs of change and for any signs that any drug is not agreeing with the patient. The nurses are the key providers of care to the patient and the family, and often also the educators of the family, showing them how to do things to help the patient. Their role is a huge one, one which can always be extended with extra qualifications or extra study, something which is becoming easier in the field of terminal care all the time.

Professional education

Standards of education and training in the field of palliative care have improved immeasurably since writing the first edition of this book. The UK government now sees it as politically important to announce extra funds for training of healthcare staff beyond cancer in palliative and terminal care (December 2003), something singularly unlikely to have happened in previous years. The issue of dying is up there on the political agenda, and, meanwhile, courses for healthcare professionals, and ethical and standards codes for professionals around death and dying, have improved immeasurably.

Macmillan Cancer Relief have piloted the Gold Standard method of training and development for primary care, whilst hospices run short courses for all kinds of health professionals and care workers. Specialist social workers in palliative and terminal care are now training others in what might be needed and useful, and the Royal Marsden Hospital and others run many courses, particularly for nurses, in caring for terminal cancer patients.

Indeed, since palliative care has become more and more of an academic specialty, and since journals are now devoted to it – as is at least one to the study of death and dying itself (*Mortality*) – the creation, delivery and monitoring of short courses has become easier. The only difficulty is getting them sufficiently targeted at the right groups, and sufficiently focused on the specific needs of a group, such as that of clergy, or volunteer sitters with dying patients, who give carers a break.

For what each of those groups needs is very different. Often, they are best able to say themselves what it is they need. But gradually courses of all kinds are being developed to meet most needs. The imperative is to make sure that those who have the needs are able to go on them, and that applies whether it is health professionals (many of whom find it difficult to get such a course paid for unless they are working directly in the field of palliative care, even though they may well need to deal with death frequently, such as those who are district nurses, GPs or social workers).

There are many profession specific courses, of which the best known and easiest to access are those basically for doctors, nurses, clergy, professions allied to medicine, and, increasingly, for funeral directors. The obvious gaps lie in training for teachers to help their pupils face death in the family or amongst their classmates on the rare occasions when it happens. There is also a need for more training in the field for social workers, many of whom have very little in their basic training and yet may need to have considerable skill and expertise when dealing with clients who have been bereaved or who have been told that they themselves are dying. Similarly, there is a need for more training for the police in this field, though in recent years that has improved considerably, since police are often the ones to have to break the news of a death to someone.

There is also considerable need for specialist training for those who provide counselling and support in a more general way, such as most forms of coun-sellors, primary care staff, GPs, and people such as hospital cleaners and ambulance staff, who all too often get ignored when it comes to this kind of training, and yet provide a great deal of support and comfort to all sorts of people facing their own death or that of a close relative.

There is another whole group of people who need help with coming to terms with what is happening, who need education and training to face their realities. These people are very often the patients themselves, who have been told that they have a terminal illness but may still have a long time to live, and their families and friends. There is a real role here for education and training in how to live with a sentence of death hanging over one's head. It is not always just a question of support and comfort. The best of counsellors and carers teach people how to make the most of life, how to live with various disabilities, how to enjoy things that seemed impossible to do again. And that area of education, because it seems more like specific personal support, has been neglected. It can come about through a support group for people with some kinds of cancer, for instance, or through a network of multiple sclerosis (MS) sufferers. It does not much matter how it comes about – it only matters that those who are working with such people realise that, as well as support, some kind of training in what to expect, how one might react, what options there are, how other people have dealt with a similar situation, is very useful.

But such support and caring takes its toll of those who give it. Those who give support to the dying people and their families also need support them-selves. Within the hospice world, that is well recognised. In the rest of the healthcare environment, it is much less common and leads to burn-out, which is a source of great sorrow to those who have admired the skill and dedica-tion of those who work day in and day out with difficult and often tragic situations.

Professionals: chaplains

Some people will want to see the priest, the counsellor, the chaplain or their own clergyperson. The question of how such a pastoral person should care for the dying person in the family is a major one, and by no means all chaplains, clergy and others get it right. Ainsworth-Smith and Speck (1982) discussed these issues in their classic work on the subject, and isolated four aspects to the pastoral task. First, the pastor can help to reconcile: that is, re-establish broken relationships between human being and human being, and between human being and God, and frequently within the patient himself. Secondly, he or she can help to support: the dying person needs support and sustenance if he or she is to endure and transcend what is happening to mind and body. Thirdly, he or she is there to guide: many people look to the clergy to guide them in what to do, in their understanding of what is happening to them, and of their faith. Fourthly, he or she can enable growth so that the dying person can, with the time that is available, use the dying process as a time of healing and spiritual growth, something which happens remarkably often.

Within these four aims, pastoral care can involve various practical 'means of grace' (in Christian terms) alongside the ongoing giving of time, support and comfort, and meaning. For some people these will involve prayer, meditation and Bible reading or reading from other holy works, depending on the faith of the individual. For others, sacramental ministry in Christianity, or other forms of sacramental rites may be required. Not all faiths have last rites, but most have rituals of devotion and attention at one's end. However, for all, it is the quality of the pastoral relationship that is most important.

Not all clergy are particularly good at this sort of ministry. Kubler-Ross and others commented on the way even the clergy will avoid dealing with the hard questions, and avoid sitting with a dying person waiting for a question that may never even be asked at all, instead of being there in case it should be – being prepared to talk about the hard things, the pain, the grief, the parting, the religious questions of life's meaning.

Even for those who are better at creating and maintaining such a personal relationship, the task is not easy. Clergy carry with them a series of complex expectations – to be able to 'answer for God', to be the bearer of the sick person's anger against God (or against the doctor, or the hospital). The fact that those providing this kind of pastoral care can often only share the pain without an 'answer' sometimes make the care of the dying one of the most demanding tasks facing the clergy or anyone who takes on this role.

Pastoral carers working within a theological framework, whatever it might be, usually have a basis for understanding the fear and rejection of death. Death has a theological significance in most, if not all, the world's religions. Death is usually the enemy. Death – with its sting – has won. Hope is ever present, but at the moment of death it seems curiously in abeyance. And belief in an afterlife is diminishing in many groups in society. So where those who are providing pastoral care really do believe in God's grace, and/or in eternal life, they are able to bring a kind of certainty of hope that many people find very comforting – even if they, as the recipients of this care, do not wholly believe what is being said themselves. It can, however, go the other way. Those more doubtful about the theological certainties can find it extremely irritating to hear from a member of the clergy a voice of certainty about, say, the afterlife, and can ask a clergy person to leave because they find it so offensive to be told a series of what they regard as platitudinous certainties, which cannot, in their own minds, make sense.

Of course, those providing pastoral care from the standpoint of a particular religious faith also bring a certain amount of ritual with them in most cases, which many dying people, whatever they actually believe, find very comforting. Social groups, whether secular or religious, tend to develop various rituals to help individuals cope with life crises and transitions. Rituals help people to come to terms with the changes that are happening in their lives. By staging the grieving process, they help people to move from one phase to another.

Funerals can provide some of this for bereaved people, and the priest, clergyman, rabbi or imam's role at the funeral involves three different aspects. The community of faith, which the priest or whoever represents, can act as a support and help to bereaved people, and indeed often does. For religious people, having death rituals set in the context of some kind of theological understanding helps give an interpretation to the death and the loss. For instance, Christianity can often help bereaved people who are Christians face the loss of death by turning the pain of bereavement into a sense of hope and confidence. The resources of the community of faith, and the support of friends, help the bereaved person make the choice between whether the death of a loved one will remain an open wound, or whether they will move towards building a new life. Going from being wife to widow can be helped by the physical and social event of the funeral, marking for her and for her friends and colleagues and fellow congregants the ending of one phase of her life and the beginning of another.

For Jews and Muslims, to name but two minorities, the support of a community which has particular ways of doing things can also be very comforting, and can help the bereaved come to terms with loss, as they do what they have to do, according to the expectations of their own particular faith group. Indeed, because in those two cases, as with other minorities, the community tends to come out and give support to bereaved people at the time of a death, the dying person and the family or friends often feel the religious community is bringing at least the hope of a kind of a future, without the dying person there, to everyone gathered round. The clergy, as the people who encourage the community to gather round and lend its support, and officiate at the rituals, whatever they might be, bring enormous support to the families.

The real problems come when someone has no religious belief (increasingly common) or belongs to a particular minority community and has done nothing about it for years, and therefore has no idea what the rituals ought to be, and has a family who are going to be bereaved who have no idea either what the rituals might be. Clergy can be very impatient with people like this, but have a lot to give in support to those who do not know what to do. More effort from religious communities and their leaders to help those who do not know the rituals to learn them, and, even more importantly, to feel comfortable with them, is urgently needed, and it is a role which the clergy could easily take on board. And it would certainly make dying, and the death rituals, easier for a great many people if that were to happen.

See Chapter 4 for further information on pastoral care and chaplains and other clergy.

Social workers and counsellors

At some stage, it may be appropriate for pastoral counsellors, and the bereavement service, if it exists, to bring together a group of bereaved people in a self-support group. For pastoral carers may eventually be able to help the grieving person set limits to their grief, and get them to begin to readjust to 'normal' life – though life may not feel 'normal' to them possibly ever again. Pastoral carers, whether they are counsellors or clergy, need to be constantly alert to the possibility that grief may become a pathological condition, so that different help may be needed from expert professionals. That is not at all uncommon, particularly in cases where there was other unresolved grief present before this particular bereavement, or where the type of loss, of a child, for instance, or as a great shock in an accident, is very difficult to get a grip on, or make any sense of – for any of us, let alone those who have to experience such horrors.

Those involved in caring for bereaved people (particularly family, but also doctors, nurses or friends) need to try and understand what is going on. If the grief becomes pathological, then specialist help must be called in, which is one reason why bereavement services, though often bereaved people say they do not want them, are so helpful. Bereavement counsellors are specially trained to pick up the signs of abnormal grieving patterns, and can often get someone referred for expert help quickly and relatively painlessly, because they know the system, and know who the best people to go to locally are.

Those helping the bereaved person, whoever they may be, have a difficult task in helping the grieving person overcome the tendencies to build abnormal defences against the pain of loss. They also have to open them up to the resources, such as bereavement counselling services, increasingly available nationwide, which will help them towards resolution of their grief. For that reason, encouraging bereaved people to go through the rituals of grieving, where they exist, is a positive benefit, to the extent that, for Christians from the Church of England, the lack of such rituals can actually be a cause of difficulty. It can be hard for pastoral carers to say to someone that there is no particular 'action' to be taken. Lighting a candle or saying formal evening prayers or not shaving or some such outward symbol often makes the grieving easier, and gives the pastoral carers a role, if they come from a faith community.

Counsellors can often help a bereaved person find a way of expressing his or her grief, even if he or she does not have a religion in which there are rituals to be performed which act as a way of channelling the expression of agony and pain. Counsellors can also often keep a weather eye on someone to see if they are making 'progress' in resolving some of the grief, so that, though no-one ever 'gets over' such a loss, they can carry on with normal life. And that is the prime role of the counsellor, be that person a professional counsellor alone, or a clergyperson, or a nurse or a doctor. For counselling is something to be provided by a variety of different professionals, and counselling skills are skills many health professionals, particularly, perhaps, people working in the field of palliative and terminal care, would do well to acquire. Increasingly, specialist courses in palliative care have a counselling element. That can be of variable quality, and a specialist counselling course dealing with dying and bereavement is often very valuable for people who work in this area, whatever their role happens to be – healthcare professional, clergy, social worker or whoever.

Social workers often work with those elderly people who are most isolated, and they can also be invaluable in working with those elderly people in nursing homes, whose need for bereavement support is often curiously unrecognised. Social workers have a key role in linking up isolated bereaved people with such services as exist for them, and, where possible, finding an entry point into some community which might be able to give some support, as well as bereavement counselling.

Getting the best out of dying – helping people die well

The dying process itself can be life-enhancing for the people who are dying, if we support them well and listen to them. But we have to achieve more than that. Suppose we manage to get it right, or nearly right, for the people who are themselves actually dying. There are at least two other groups to be considered. First comes the family, the about to be widow or widower or children or siblings – whoever the nearest and dearest are. They will certainly need our support, though almost all of healthcare training has suggested to us that it is the patient who should be the primary focus of our attention. Nevertheless, if we are caring for dying people, then their families and friends become part of the package too. Their relationships with family and friends become so important, affect so profoundly what they feel, that to ignore everyone except the patient would be foolish. That does not mean that medical details would, necessarily, be discussed with anyone else but the patient, unless the individual was unable to participate in decision making any longer. But it does mean that the family and friends have to be kept informed, at least in rough outline, that they may have to take decisions, at least in part, in consultation with the health professionals, if and when the dying person becomes incapable. And health staff have a particular role in trying to do everything they can to prevent the atmosphere of dishonesty that can grow up between a couple, or between a parent and a child. One says that the dying person is not terminally ill (it can be either the patient or the member of the family most concerned) and the other either colludes or feels uncomfortable with contradicting. That way, through a lack of honesty, in the mistaken belief that not telling will mean people feeling better about things (when all the evidence suggests that they feel worse), lies intense, confusing and harder nursing when the dying person is no longer capable of making decisions for him- or herself.

So the encouragement of honesty, and the keeping informed in broad outline, are essential parts of caring for a dying person and their family. That attitude, properly managed with the encouragement of honesty and the push to settle outstanding scores, to talk about anything on people's minds, the encouragement to talk about deep feelings, can make the process of dying life-enhancing for the person who is actually terminally ill and for the members of the family who find that this period of dying brings them closer together and allows a lot of unfinished business to be dealt with. Health professionals can be very good at bringing people together and encouraging them to talk about things that matter. After all, there is not necessarily much time left.

But, of course, time is of the essence. Though there is not much time left, the dying person often wants to be given the illusion that there is plenty of time. If it is healthcare professionals, the idea that they are rushing about, unable to sit and talk to a dying man or woman, is anathema both to that person and to his or her family and friends. What the dying person often wants of us is time. Similarly, if we are the family and friends, most of us are busy, busy, all day long. Making space and time for our dying parents or relatives is hard in the extreme. We do not have the time to do it. We cannot predict accurately enough when the person is going to die to book ourselves a week's holiday in order to be there. We try to do everything at once, and we become stressed and distressed. Yet we need the time. The dying person needs the time.

It is worth thinking about how we can achieve this. Some hospices have a rule that one day a week is a no-visitor day, to give the relatives a break. Similarly, those of us trying to combine being there with the dying person and a job and other family responsibilities must be kind to ourselves where we can, and take time off, give ourselves a break, read, listen to the radio, watch TV, go for a walk, talk to our spouses. It has to be done so that the whole process for the dying person does not feel as if we are all in a rush, with no time to stop and stare and talk and share. So those of us who are caring for the dying person, whether as professional healthcare workers, doctors, nurses, physiotherapists and so on, or as family members, have to relax our pace. The dying person has not got much time left. He or she wants our time, our calm. We need to give it to them. That means slowing our pace, and being prepared to pace ourselves as well.

For dying people will often say, once they know the prognosis, that they are delighted because they have a little more time. We need to help them use it properly, as they want to. And that we cannot do by arriving in a rush, rushing off, or, as nurses, skipping past the bed or the room, unable to stop the usual tasks of a busy healthcare setting.

For what does the dying person want of us? Often to talk, quietly. To listen. To read poetry. To share with us intimate thoughts, often expressed with great difficulty. That last time, those few last weeks and hours, are not to be rushed. But we need to let the dying person value the little time they have left, by treating them to much of our time, sharing with them what they have. Listening, talking, encouraging.

But there is one other group who should be able to get something out of caring for the dying – the health professionals. Caring for dying people should be life-enhancing for them. Often it is. The experience of hospice care has made it clear that, with considerable support from psychologists and counsellors (often much needed), staff find the work they do enormously enriching. But support for staff so that they can talk about their emotions to someone who will not mind, who will not judge them harshly for having needed to do it, is essential. If caring for dying people is to be done well, then health professionals involved in that care need to be supported in their work. That support can come from professional counsellors, or from volunteers who will give their time to hear what the professionals have to say. Professional counsellors and psychologists are infinitely preferable, because the relationship of professional to professional is easier to manage. But that support is vital if those who are working with the dying are themselves to gain good things from their work, and are to give the most they can, the best they can, to what they do. After all, they are caring for people at the end of their lives, in intense emotional and spiritual circumstances in many cases. The nearest and dearest to the bereaved will remember for the rest of their days what happened at that point. The professionals want to do it well. But the stress in doing it well, in not switching off from intense emotion, is considerable. And that stress has to be dealt with to allow the professionals to carry on doing a supportive, caring job.

For palliative care is more than pain relief. It is about encouraging dying people and their families to live life to the full insofar as is possible in the circumstances. It is about completing the personal and inter-personal agenda. It is about trying to make sure that there is no unfinished business. Professionals can help that along very considerably, but only with support themselves. For it is professionals who can encourage those who are dying and their families and friends to face things head on, on the basis that nothing is so bad if we know what it is. But encouraging people to look death square in the eyes, think about its implications, and set things to rights in this world, is hard, emotionally stressful, exhausting work. If we are all to get the best out of this final experience in this life, we must not only look after our patients and their relatives and friends, but our healthcare professionals as well.

Who takes the lead?

Part of the recipe for that clearly lies in giving our health professionals a considerable amount of good support, both formal and informal. But there is another way we can help to get the best kind of death for those we care for, or for ourselves if we are the patients. And that is by deciding who takes the lead in the team of people who have to create the environment for dying well. For the obvious leader, the person to set the tone, the pace, to make the demands and so on, is the person who is dying him- or herself. But that is only possible up to a point. Some people, albeit very ill and taking a considerable amount of pain killing drugs, will have a mind clear as a bell, and be quite capable not only of saying what it is they want and do not want, but also setting the emotional temperature for it all. But that is comparatively rare. What tends to happen is that the person who is dying begins by setting the lead, begins to say what it is he or she wants, makes it clear about the level of honesty required (often helped by the health professionals, especially nurses, who find dishonesty, these days, hard to deal with), and then reaches a stage where clarity begins to go. Or, if not clarity, more often than not the energy to make a case and fight for it begins to elude dying people. In those circumstances, several things need to happen.

First, the health professionals need to be certain that they have made a note of what the individual wanted before this stage of lack of clarity or energy occurs. They need to have that note easily accessible. Secondly, a meeting often needs to be held of the professionals and the family to discuss what was wanted by the person concerned when they found it easier to express those sorts of ideas. The professionals need to make it very clear at this stage that they feel under a bounden, professional, duty to stick with those desires. Families sometimes want to change things on the basis that 'Uncle Sam would not have wanted that if he was in his right mind'. But, if Uncle Sam did not want it, he had every opportunity to say so. Professional staff have the advantage of not having the same emotional involvement, the same emotional baggage, however emotionally draining this kind of patient can be. The professional can know what the patient wanted, and can make it clear to the family and friends that that was the case.

In this situation, the second requirement for the professionals is that they very clearly take the lead. They are, in that sense, in charge. The patient, whilst he or she can, sets the pace. From then on it becomes a team effort, between patient, professionals and family and friends. But the professionals, whenever there is any difficulty about what the right course of action might be, must take the lead. In the team of carers, including the patient him- or herself, the professional becomes the leader once the patient cannot manage to set the agenda sufficiently firmly any longer.

This requires immense strength on the part of the professionals, for families, friends and spouses of the patients can be extraordinarily demanding and difficult. But this is where the professional can truly sit or stand on his or her professional dignity and status. The message often needs to be 'I am in charge round here, and I decide what happens', as firmly as that. But that is the nature of professional leadership, all too often required when caring for dying patients. And the trick is to retain the leadership position, whilst making all the other members of the team feel that they are playing a full part and contributing to the decision-making process. For the best kind of care for a dying person is when everyone feels that they are making a really useful contribution, where they feel they can all discuss what is best, acknowledging that the dying person him- or herself must say what is wanted. But the trick for professionals is to take the lead over members of the dying person's family and their friends whilst including them in the caring – it is by virtue of doing that that the healthcare professionals can set up a true team spirit amongst the carers, and manage to make the dying good and sustaining, and the caring process sustaining and uplifting as well. Indeed, the example of how caring for people with AIDS has been handled, with 'buddies' who befriend the person with AIDS and teams of volunteers doing a variety of tasks is not a bad model for providing really good quality care, and really supportive emotional care, for a dying person, according to their wishes, as long as those are clear.

Family members

It is very hard to be in the least prescriptive for family members of bereaved people, because families work in such very different ways. Some want to cling closely together, whilst others prefer to experience their deepest emotions more privately, though the family will come and give the bereaved person a great deal of attention. But there are basic things families can do, including looking out for some of the signs of abnormal grief mentioned above.

Some of those things are obvious, such as ensuring the person who is bereaved actually eats properly. It is extraordinary how many bereaved people report an appalling loss of appetite, and having lost some 15 pounds around my father's death, although I was aware that one has to eat, I am convinced that for bereaved people knowing that they 'have to eat' is no great help – they need to be encouraged to do so. The easiest way is when food is brought to them and put on a plate in front of them. That is why, no doubt, so many religious groups and various cultures have a ritual of mourning which includes bringing particular foods and encouraging the mourners to eat. Indeed, most groups have a tradition of some kind which includes bringing food to the house of mourning, no doubt because it is a universal human (and animal) trait, to stop eating, not to notice the pressure of hunger, when grieving. And so the first thing for any family member to do is to ensure that the bereaved person or people are eating.

Secondly, it is important to ensure that the bereaved people go out and back into the 'real world' as soon as the culture or religious group expects it. In other words, the natural tendency of many bereaved people is to stay at home, particularly because they do not want to have to meet people and talk about the person who has died. Or, even worse, go out and find that they are not doing so, because neighbours and friends avoid the subject, making pain which is searing even worse. Family members can play an important role in encouraging the bereaved person to go out again, and indeed in taking them out.

Thirdly, they can ensure that the bereaved person is not left alone too much. People vary enormously in how much they want to be alone. But it is important that bereaved people, though one cannot alleviate their loneliness, for it is a particular loneliness to do with the person they have lost, are not alone too much, and are encouraged to go out and do the ordinary things of life again.

Fourthly, it is important to help bereaved people over the 'first' birthday, or Christmas, or Jewish New Year, or Id, or whatever it may be, after the death. The first one is often very painful. It brings back all kinds of memories, often dredging up thoughts which have not been in the bereaved person's mind for decades. And it is very important that they have company at those particular times.

There are many other things that family members can do. The most important thing to be aware of, however, is that bereaved people behave in very different ways from each other, and it is hard to predict how they will behave when it comes to it. So what family members have to do is play everything at the pace that the bereaved person sets, and be prepared to provide help and support at that pace, in that way. Families are probably the best source of support and help there is for bereaved people, other than the specialist and highly skilled support of healthcare professionals. So it is important that family members, and friends, think hard about how to do it. It is a mixture of doing what comes naturally and thinking hard about how to do it in order to cause no offence, and to get the best effect.

But, long before helping the bereaved person, families are usually very involved in helping with the person who is dying. There is some evidence to suggest that people live longer if they have family to support them and to live for, including family events such as the birth of a grandchild or a family wedding. Families tend to forget family rifts when someone is dying too, because there is no time left to sort it out, and many people report huge satisfaction from helping to care for a family member. However, it does have to be said that there is some evidence that it is better to be a man who dies at home tended by a wife and family. My mother, when my father died, asked 'Who looks after the women?'. The answer is the children, but they rarely live with the surviving parent, usually female. And they have their own, often very busy, lives to lead. But families do care for their own. Young and Cullen (1996) report that it would certainly be better to be the elderly head of a large and traditional family to get the best kind of family care. Nevertheless, they also report an estranged sister coming back from Australia to be with her brother, and various other family reunions. But it is the traditional families where it is easiest. Someone is there to care. The other family members support the carer, and come and see the person who is dying all the time. And relief for the carer can be provided by other family members, as well as by a hospice or such like. It is clear that those families whose origins are in the Indian sub-continent or in Ireland or in eastern Europe still often have the structures that make all this work better. Health professionals often make assumptions that, in those kinds of families, there is little for them to do. That may be the case, but, equally, I have often heard people from precisely those backgrounds saying that, when it came to it, however wonderful in a way it is to be part of a particular structure and way of doing things, it can become oppressive, and you are not allowed simply to follow your own inclinations in how to grieve and show your loss. So, despite the obvious advantages of large, extended, supportive families, there can be disadvantages too, and we need to watch out for them.

However, traditional or not, families do still care for their own very considerably. Despite everything that has been said about families not providing care, all the evidence about carers, about people providing 20 hours of care a week as well as working full-time, suggests that caring in Britain is alive and well and provided largely, but by no means wholly, by women. And people who are dying, on the whole, but not always, prefer to be looked after at home, although there are many people who prefer the most intimate functions, such as toileting, to be carried out by a professional rather than a family member.

Communities

In many urban areas, close-knit communities, as we once understood them, have disappeared except for minority ethnic groups. Thus, whilst you may have a close community of Bangladeshis in Tower Hamlets, you are less likely to have a close community of old East End dockers. They have partly moved away; they tend not to know their Bangladeshi neighbours, more because of language problems than racism, and they tend to be more linked into family than neighbours.

But, though that seems to be more and more the pattern in the inner city, there are many exceptions. Certainly, in many areas, neighbours are wonderful. Particularly if people have lived in the same area for a long time, neighbours will tend to be on the alert, looking to see how things are going when one of their neighbours that they know is ill. Similarly, in more rural areas, neighbours and the wider community can be marvellous. There are countless stories of neighbours and friends taking people from a rural village to a hospital for treatment, and indeed, doing all the transporting as the treatment leaves the patient feeling weaker and weaker.

The worst area for community feeling tends to be the outer suburbs of big cities and the suburban, stockbroker-belt type areas. People have more space, so they tend to know less by observation of what is going on with their neighbours. There is also less community spirit generally, and, apart from local groups such as church or social groups (the golf club, for instance) people can live very isolated lives.

For that reason, the community can be less than supportive at the time someone is dying, unless that person belongs to a particular organisation or religious community, or is well-known for some other reason. But there is still a great tradition of neighbours helping. In Michael Young's and Lesley Cullen's *A Good Death*, two of their 14 interviewees were largely cared for by neighbours, and that was in an area of east London where old-style neighbourliness was said to be on the way out.

And, when Deborah Moggach's partner of 10 years standing, the well-known cartoonist Mel Calman, died at her side in a cinema, very suddenly, she wrote about her experiences in *The Times*. Amongst many of the other things she wrote about, was the support of friends, the people who came clutching a bottle of vodka and lunch, the countless people who rang, the people who came and filled her fridge. She wrote how she was asked all the time if she had hit the bottle yet, but explained that she could not because every time she stretched out her hand, the phone rang. Meanwhile her sister came and stayed at nights, slipping away in the morning, and friends came round, and talked about Mel.

That has to be right. Social networks, our friends and neighbours and families, have in the end to be our prime sources of support. Everything ever said against retired people moving away to live in a place they do not know, where the local people do not know them, has to be borne in mind here. For, if one of a couple dies, the other is left isolated. Far better to stay in the old home, in the old area, and know that, when the time comes, and one needs help, it will be there. For old friends, family and neighbours come up trumps. In the 11 weeks after my father died, as I was first writing this, my mother did not have a day when someone did not ask her out and come to visit – quite apart from family. The role of one's wider support network is never so clearly defined as in bereavement, and often whilst someone is dying. But we write about it, think about it, describe it, all too rarely.

Certainly, other anecdotes and personal experiences lead me to think that neighbours are still very good in many circumstances. Our experience when my father died was that neighbours were wonderful whilst he was so ill, and that after his death the support they gave my mother was quite wonderful, and continuing. Instead of all the old stories about kindness after a death lasting only a couple of weeks, my mother and other bereaved people I have known often said that people are wonderful for months and indeed years.

But, there is undoubtedly more that communities can do, and indeed more that those who are dying and those who care for them can do, to encourage them to do it. For instance, if a person who is dying was or is a member of a religious group, then the carers can let the leader of that group (the clergy-man, the priest, the imam, the rabbi) know about the situation and encourage visits and support. Similarly, if the person was active in a political group, the secretary of the local Labour or Liberal Democrat constituency party or Conservative Association can be telephoned and told of what is happening. That applies to the golf club, to the Women's Institute, to the Townswomen's Guild, and so on. Most organisations, if they are told of someone's troubles and that they are dying, will help. There is a considerable human desire to be helpful, even if there is embarrassment about knowing what to do.

Health professionals can often help here. If there is embarrassment, they can suggest particular things to the organisation concerned. They can suggest visits, or shopping, sitting to give the carer a break, taking someone out in a wheelchair if they have a car which is suitable, and so on. Most people, if something practical and well within their capabilities is suggested, agree with alacrity, but it would still be a help if local churches and other organisations were to set up groups precisely to help members of the group who are sick and dying, because there is a way people can learn by experience to be even more helpful, and can learn some of the basic skills about lifting and touching someone painfully thin and very weak. It would be a real bonus if churches and other organisations took that on board, perhaps getting very basic training from a local hospice or homecare team. Indeed, it is the obvious next step from the fundraising many local organisations of all kinds do for their local hospice and homecare team.

Society

Society is really just a group of communities. Society at large has become much better at dealing with dying people and the bereaved than it was in the 1960s and 1970s. The hospice movement has provided a tremendous fillip to those who want to be able to talk about how they wish to die, and the growth of bereavement services, even if it is because of the decline in traditional family and friendship patterns, and the decline in active church going, has made talking about bereavement, and seeking help when feeling desperate after a bereavement, entirely respectable.

What society has to do now is to bring itself to talk more openly about the good death. Instead of conversations being about euthanasia, which is illegal, though discussions are taking place in Parliament about it, yet again, as I write this second edition, more conversations should be about how we want to die, and where, who we want at our bedside when it comes to it, and what kind of funeral we want. Society can encourage that kind of discussion, and society can allow people to talk openly about their grief, instead of covering it up.

More than all this, however, society has to think about how it wants to allow people to grieve, how it wishes to encourage not only open discussion of grief, but time and space for grieving, through more compassionate leave, perhaps, or through time off for support groups, or simply by encouraging people who are grief-stricken to return to work even if they cannot yet concentrate on what they are doing. And the role of friends and neighbours at the time of a death is so crucial that employers and others need to think, society as a whole needs to think, about how we allow the time to people to comfort the mourner. This should not only be part of religious traditions, but something we expect of neighbours and friends, part of what society expects of people, a bit like giving blood.

Society has a role in encouraging better funerals, and in insisting that dying happens with dignity, funerals happen with dignity (perhaps taking longer than the 20 minutes allocated at the crematorium), and that grief in bereavement is something people should be encouraged to express to others, who should also learn how to reply, how to respond, and how, silently, to proffer support. Early signs are there, but there is clearly a large piece of work for society to do, to talk through, to think through, to encourage ways of acknowledging grief, ways of comforting the broken hearted, that can become part of a norm without necessarily being a part of a religious or cultural tradition. We need to be able to say: 'I recognise your grief' as easily as we say: 'How are you?', so that it becomes what society does to support those who have lost a loved one, and what society does to give comfort – even though we no longer walk around with black armbands or any other outward sign. And perhaps we need to reinvent the wearing of mourning or some other outward sign to help society behave differently to those who are mourning, and bereaved – a new social statement that helps people get along together better, especially when times are hard for some individuals.

As well as this, much more could be done in the field of education for the general public around death and dying. Just as there needs to be education for parenting, and education to enable young people to deal with many of the ordinary things of life, some discussion of death and dying is useful when children are still at school. This is for several reasons. First, there is a strong argument, when we no longer see our dead relatives at home, and are drawn into the death of grandparents and so on, for children to be taught something of what happens, something of how we care for dying people in our society.

Many schools already have a relationship with a local hospice, and the young people go in and talk to some of the patients and their families, or raise money for the hospice. In that case, the relationship with death and dying is entirely natural. But, all too often, a child at school will be thrown by the death of a grandparent, where teachers will not know how involved or not the child has been, and will not necessarily know how close they were, or how upset the child is. When it is the first death a young person has seen, it is almost always very upsetting, and getting back to 'normal' can take quite a long time. Young people grieve, but they may not show it as older people do, nor as small children do either, and they may also be embarrassed at showing how much they miss a grandparent – often, it is thought a bit 'wet' or pathetic to make a fuss about the loss of a grandparent, when most young people would sympathise very considerably with the death of a parent.

Indeed, since it is likely that in almost every class of children there will be a loss, probably in fact of a grandparent but also, not uncommonly, of a parent, it is important that the young people be given the chance to discuss the meaning of death (which will vary considerably according to the religion and social group from which they come) and the actual events surrounding the death. For many young people, the first funeral they have ever gone to is that of a member of the family, often someone very close indeed. Some knowledge at least of what happens at a funeral, what sorts of prayers are said, what people do afterwards, and something about tombstones, cemeteries and crematoria, at the most basic, can be quite helpful

Clearly this is partly a matter for personal and social education (PSE) teachers, but it also comes into religious studies. Indeed, death and dying can be one of those cross-disciplinary themes which can unite a school in a strange way. English lessons can be focused on poetry about death and novels with a good description of a deathbed scene. History can focus on some battlefield deaths or on the untimely end of a great hero or villain. Religious studies can focus on the meaning of death in many different religions, and PSE can look at what death means to the young people concerned and how it is dealt with in our society at present.

At the moment, death and dying are rarely on the syllabus for any young people at school. Yet there is a strong argument for it to be, and, perhaps, an argument for saying it should be, particularly because it is so little discussed in most homes. And, if it were more widely discussed, we might be better at dealing with our own dying and that of our nearest and dearest when the time comes.

4

The best that we can do

Sources of support

Religious and pastoral care

There is a relatively low rate of attendance at places of worship in Britain, such that only some 16% of the population attend services two or three times monthly, compared with 43% in the USA, 78% in the Irish Republic and 58% in Northern Ireland. Similarly, only 64% are affiliated with a religious denomination, compared with 93% in the USA, 98% in the Irish Republic and 92% in Northern Ireland.[1] It might therefore seem to be surprising that a very high proportion of those who die (it was 95% according to Argyle and Beit-Hallahmi in 1975, and I have been unable to find a later figure) have a religious funeral. This is, of course, partly due to the fact that when there is a death in the family, everyone has the right to ask the priest of their parish to officiate, whatever their faith, and there are always duty clergy at crematoria. A parish priest can say no if he or she does not feel that the person was a Christian, but in fact, on the whole, anyone who wants a Christian funeral, conducted by the parish priest or the duty clergyman at a crematorium, can have one. The high rate of those who want religious funerals is also because people find it very difficult to have a funeral that is 'non-religious', because there is on the whole an absence of words, though there is an increasing occurrence of cremations, especially, held after the death of someone who had no faith at all, where friends come together to say good things about the person who has died (*de mortuis nihil nisi bonum* – nothing about the dead unless it is good – seems to apply in all varieties of funeral). And people from minority religious traditions and cultures often want a funeral in accordance with that religion even if they were 'lapsed' in their lives.

When discussing the somewhat out-of-date survey figures quoted above Argyle and Beit-Hallahmi commented: 'It looks as if, in Britain today, religion is seen by many people primarily as a means of dealing with death'. One might add to that both birth and, where it occurs, marriage, which is still flourishing despite our massive divorce rate. But certainly religious organisations are 'used' by those of little faith all too frequently for great life events. In my view, there is no reason why they should not be, and indeed I think it churlish of clergy of all religions and denominations to be so reluctant to officiate at life events for people who have not hitherto been active. After all, it might be a way of getting people involved in the religious life of the community, and as most religious organisations are reporting a fall in attendance one might have thought that encouraging people to come by being willing to help them at a life crisis or even an ordinary life event, such as marriage, would be sensible.

Certainly, there is frequently an increase in religious attitudes and feelings as people get older, despite the fact that church or synagogue or mosque attendance diminishes with increasing age. That in itself has to be seen alongside people from religious minority communities, whose attendance at places of worship is much higher than the British average, even in old age, where the surrounding community will make efforts to get their older people to church, mosque, or synagogue. Indeed, questions need to be asked about whether minority communities actually go to their place of worship (which is often a community centre as well, as in the case of the gurdwara for Sikhs, or the synagogue buildings for Jews, for instance) for religious reasons in the main, or whether, sometimes, it is not rather out of a sense of identification with their community. Nevertheless, there are often difficulties for orthodox Jews attending their synagogues on sabbaths and festivals as they get older because, if they cannot walk, they are still not allowed to drive or be driven, since it is regarded as 'work' which is forbidden on the sabbath. That would only change if an eruv, technically a courtyard, which means forming an enclosed space, is declared in a town or part of a town. A battle raged for years recently in north-west London over whether areas of the Hampstead Garden Suburb could be turned into an eruv, with opponents to the scheme drawn from the Jewish community as much as the non-Jewish, and those in favour simply unable to understand the strength of feeling against. However, unless there is an eruv, it is very difficult for orthodox Jews to manage to get to synagogue at all on sabbaths and festivals if they need help in the shape of a wheelchair or to be driven by car.

It is also worth remembering that, despite relatively low church attendance figures (and at other places of worship for other faiths) there is still a relatively high degree of some form of religious faith in Britain. To quote the British Social Attitudes Survey again, 69% of people claim to believe in God (as against 94% in the USA and 95% in Ireland, north and south. More remarkably, perhaps, 55% of people believe in life after death (though quite what they mean by that is unclear), compared with 78% in the USA and Northern Ireland and 80% in the Irish Republic.[1] It is also worth saying that those percentages are higher amongst older people, and drop off with younger people who were surveyed. In other words, though conventional religion may not have a high rate of adherence in terms of 'belonging' or church attendance, people have quite strong beliefs, which are likely to manifest themselves in various ways around the time of a death, both in terms of coping with dying and in terms of dealing with the funeral and bereavement.

But, despite the relatively high level of faith of some sort, chaplains are often not the first port of call. Sometimes, people will talk to doctors and nurses. But, in hospitals particularly, rather than in hospices or in the community, some of those important conversations, some of that 'listening', for that is what it often is, is done not by doctors and nurses, but by cleaners and porters. Cleaners who have worked for years in one healthcare institution know where people are likely to talk to them and when, and look out for it. For many of them, it is the chance to have these conversations, the reward that that kind of intimacy brings, that encourages them to put up with poor pay and, often, less than good working conditions. Those who have devotedly listened and counselled over the years are often far more skilled than any of our professional counsellors, for they speak, and listen, from a wealth of ordinary, practical experience. Their listening is profoundly kind. Their advice, when it is given, is profoundly sensible. They are the people who will say: 'You must tell your daughter, or your son'. They are the ones who recognise where doubts lie, and who see patients lying, their faces turned to the wall, as King Hezekiah did when he thought he was about to die (II Kings 20:1–2), and try to help, albeit very quietly. And they are also the ones who bring the chaplain when they think it necessary, or tell the nursing staff, or simply tip a word to a member of the family.

But, despite the anecdotal evidence suggesting that cleaning staff are often very good at this, it should not be left only to them, though giving them some recognition for the support they give, and training to help them do it better, would be a good beginning. It is also unlikely that chaplains will be able to provide all the support that might be needed, or that they would have enough time to do much more than walk around and chat briefly to individual patients, which is an argument for others receiving training in how to listen, and how to help, which chaplains, amongst others, might be well placed to provide. Clearly, from evidence presented at the original Derby Body and Soul conference[2] in 1996, and from the subsequent Body and Soul conferences, as well as elsewhere, nurses are being asked about spiritual matters. Clearly, too, it is all too frequently that doctors are asked about spiritual things – though very often they will not recognise the question, and instead will think it a question about the actual condition, rather than about the meaning of life.

There is a further problem. Some attitudes to healthcare are so scientifically driven, as indeed they should be because carrying out healthcare which is not scientifically valid would also be immoral, that there is little room for the human. Doctors who are trained in hi-tech medical care have often had no training in dealing with the hard questions – even with 'Am I going to die, doctor?', let alone 'What was it all for?'. To add to that, many medical students may deliberately have chosen the hi-tech specialties in order not to have the difficult questions to deal with, leaving that to the psychiatrists, though often they do not have time for it, and the GPs, who can be wonderful at it if their inclination lies that way. Yet the drive for scientific evidence makes pastoral care seem somehow pointless, or expensive, or meaningless, where, in fact, for many patients it adds meaning, and may improve the quality of their experience of healthcare, even if it does not enable them to get better physically more quickly. For, after all, with the very elderly and the terminally ill, many of them are not going to get better. What they will do is eventually die well or less well, comfortably or less comfortably, reassured or less reassured, with dignity or without. And it is those questions about how people face their end that are all too scarce in the syllabus of medical and nursing students to this very day, despite the vast popularity of the hospice movement. And it is the pastoral care which they should expect to give which is so sadly missing.

It used to be argued that healthcare professionals should give this kind of pastoral care because what they were doing was a 'vocation', a calling, like going into a religious order. Christians, particularly, see the history of medicine in the hospices of the Crusades (which have a sinister implication for Jews and Muslims) and in the great healthcare institutions that were church founded (St Thomas' Hospital, St Bartholomew's Hospital) and taken over only too recently by the state. Add to that the undoubtedly Christian thinking behind the great Victorian philanthropists who set up the poor hospitals and the lying-in hospitals, the work of Florence Nightingale, herself being driven by a passionate Christianity of a kind, and one can see where the idea of the religious vocation for healthcare professionals came from.

But, even if it were once true, it is not so now. People are professional healthcare workers, whether doctors or nurses or physiotherapists or the like. Some will have religious feelings. Some will even be driven in some of what they do by altruism. But one cannot demand a vocational call for them. Instead, we should demand the highest standards, and the greatest empathy and sympathy for those they care for. Included in that empathy should be a form of pastoral care, or at least a recognition that pastoral care can be helpful.

But, if there is a clergyman, priest or religious leader who has had pastoral contact with a family over many months or years, he or she may well be better able to have some of those conversations in detail, and will very likely be the first to be called when someone is diagnosed as being terminally ill. In the non-religious, so-called Church of England majority (thus described because of how they fill in a form when asked their religious allegiance, as 'C of E', rather than any statement of actual belief), even for those who have no formal religious allegiance, and who do not meet the clergyman until they see him at the crematorium door, it is still widely believed that there is something appropriate about the minister being 'involved' at the time of death. Somehow it is 'part of his job'. He or she is necessary for disposing of the physical remains, and it is a proper role for anyone who takes a leadership position in a religious organisation, so that it can be the case, say, in a small Jewish community where there is no rabbi, for a lay member of the congregation to conduct the service. That is appropriate, because they are acting, for that purpose, as religious leaders.

Where people do have religious faith, however, the religious leader has often had a longer, more continuous relationship with a person than almost any other professional 'helper', although, increasingly, a GP or district nurse who takes long-term care of an individual, can have as long a relationship as a clergyman, with many of the same pastoral elements within the pattern of care. There is a growing sense in religious groupings in Britain that there cannot, need not, always be a professional religious leader. There is a growing rediscovery of the personal and pastoral benefits of belonging to a caring community, though 'community care' is seen as often meaning little or no care when used in the sense of discharge from long-stay institutions.

In Christianity, the priest or clergyperson is supposed to have a vocation to provide a caring relationship. That is less true of other religious groups, where there is a stronger sense of the whole community caring for everyone within that community. Whilst the imam or rabbi might set the lead, and, indeed, as a result of Christian influence and example about the idea of 'ministry', might do much of the tending and caring him- or herself, in many cases there is an individual or group within the congregation charged with the responsibility for visiting the sick (bikkur cholim, visiting the sick, in Judaism, is often the responsibility of a smaller grouping of people who have a special interest in visiting the ill within the community, in hospital or at home, which is fulfilling one of the commandments in the Torah, to care for the sick).

The pastoral task for all the healthcare professionals and clergy dealing with and looking after terminally ill people, entails offering support, comfort, and meaning (no small task) to patients at times of change and crisis. The deep concerns about life's meaning or lack of it which many people feel at the time of death are real, not imagined, and healthcare professionals and those offering pastoral care within a healthcare system have to recognise that fact and not pretend that such concerns and fears are merely symptoms of something else, and call it depression. For people are right to be worried about their forthcoming death. Coming to the end of one's life is a time for assessment and reassessment. Many of us are too busy to do much assessment at any other time of our lives. It is no surprise therefore that one faces one's oncoming death with less than equanimity. It may not make us easier to deal with for the healthcare staff. It may mean that our pastoral carers, clergy and others, feel that we are not doing the right thing and confessing our sins and turning to death with 'calm of mind, all passion spent' (Milton: *Samson Agonistes*). But it is actually a reflection of how many of us feel.

There are also those amongst us who challenge healthcare professionals and clergy quite viciously as we face our deaths. We challenge their faith – in God, in the value of healthcare (after all, we are the non-successes of health-care's miraculous interventions), and then, damn it all, because we are angry, we will not even do the decent thing and die with dignity and grace. Instead, here we are, making a fuss. One hears this complaint from clergy and health-care workers all the time. Someone who is terminally ill is 'making a fuss'. The question that comes to mind then is: 'Why shouldn't they? Why shouldn't we make a fuss?' After all, how much more fuss are we going to be able to make? And, of course, according to the lights of medical science, in which we were encouraged to put our trust, for it can work miracles, we are failures. You, the medical professionals, have failed us, even though we campaigned for more research money, entered all your clinical trials, believed you when you said the chemotherapy had a good chance of working. But you gave us the chemotherapy because you did not want to admit to us that there was nothing you could do. The inability to admit defeat on the part of medical science has led to some of our anger. And when the clergy are working in that healthcare setting, they are collaborating with a system that allows us to be hoodwinked. If I had known, I would have gone on a world cruise, rather than put myself through the pain and misery and sickness.

I am only citing an example of what one hears in the pastoral setting. But what I am citing is not unusual. Healthcare professionals are often felt by dying patients to have conned them in some way. Clergy in the healthcare setting (other than a hospice, where the knowledge is there, and the die is cast) are seen as trying to maintain cheerfulness when it is simply inap-propriate. There seems to be a conspiracy that prevents anyone talking to the patient about fear, and regret, and lack of confidence in how he or she will be judged at the end of days, if that is what the patient believes is to come.

So, clergy in a hospital setting, chaplains of any kind, and health profes-sionals who are providing pastoral care of some kind, willingly or otherwise, have a hard task to perform. Those involved in this kind of care are also amongst the few in Britain who are permitted to break through the taboos associated with death. In the care of the dying and the bereaved, they have a very particular role. The clergy themselves represent the community of faith or the minority community defined by a religious label, even if not all members of that community actually have a strong religious faith as Chris-tians would understand it. They can, therefore, in the name of the church, Jewish community or Muslim community or whichever religious grouping, as a caring community, take the initiative towards people in their times of family crisis. The clergy, or even the healthcare professional if they handle it very sensitively, can bring people who are dying back into contact with their wider community, which can be enormously useful. The dying person then goes back to 'belonging' before they finally die, and their families feel happier because they have a particular way to behave at the time of the actual death which is governed by the ritual of the religion concerned.

But, that requires very careful handling. It is not the right thing to do to put a person back in touch with his or her faith because the pastoral carer (the chaplain, the nurse, the doctor) somehow feels that is the best or easiest thing to do. It has to be done because the person him- or herself wants it to happen. People who are dying must be allowed to make their own choices. The fact that healthcare workers and clergy often feel inadequate facing someone who is terminally ill, and feel that 'they would be better off with their own', is no reason for them to go ahead and make contacts. Contact has to happen with permission – more than that, with desire. It has to happen because the dying person wants it. And most dying people, if asked, will have quite clear views about what it is they want and do not want. The problem for them is the frequency with which assumptions are made about what they ought to want, but, in fact, do not.

Rituals

If such an intervention, such contact, with the religious faith is wanted, it can bring great comfort and resolution. In Christianity, for instance, the clergy person can administer the resources of 'grace' which can bring emotional, as well as spiritual, sustenance. In other faiths, the resolution, emotional and spiritual, may come about in other ways, but a discussion of the issues and concerns which divide one member of a family from another, often in the area of belief, can be very helpful, even if the only point reached is an agreement to disagree over such issues as, say, the afterlife, or the nature of Heaven and Hell. The religious leader can discuss handling guilt through forgiveness, atonement and other methods, such as fasting in some faiths. Those offering pastoral care in the healthcare setting can offer the rituals of religious practice as a way of coping with uncertainty and change – even if the meaning of each of those rituals is lost on the person who is dying. That is a very important point. The fact that people do not necessarily understand why they are carrying out some ritual, such as for instance lighting candles on the sabbath in Judaism, does not mean that carrying it out does not bring supreme comfort. In Christianity, clergy are often very shocked when one discusses the value of rituals without their symbolism necessarily being understood or even made explicit. If I explain the lighting of the sabbath candles as a way of ensuring that the individual has light to enjoy the sabbath, when the lighting of lights and fires is forbidden once the sabbath has begun, anyone but an observant Jew would argue that that was not relevant to him or her. After all, he or she will use the electric light happily. In a hospital or hospice, or at home, if bedridden and being cared for by others, the lights will be switched on anyway. What possible significance can lighting the sabbath candles then have? The answer lies in many things – in an atavistic longing for the rituals carried out by parents and grandparents and generations of forebears one never knew, in actually giving shape to a week that has distressingly little shape, as sickness leads to timelessness, leading to a fear that 'next week I'll be dead', to a sense that lighting the sabbath candles is a beacon of light in a harsh world, generally and person-ally, and a sign of hope. All of those are meanings the individual may ascribe to such a ritual. Interpreting the ritual is the patient's business; the 'real' reason may well be meaningless, yet carrying out the ritual assumes enormous importance.

The value of having rituals to help us find 'something to do' in times of great stress and pain is often something all too apparent when caring for dying people, and those healthcare professionals involved can often helpfully ask whether there is any ritual which it would be helpful for the individual patient or members of the family to perform, and can even help find resources to make it possible, such as a separate room for prayer. Even those who have not prayed in their lives, as far as they can remember, are often keen to try to pray, or contemplate, if they can, as they face their deaths, and we are horrify-ingly bad at providing physical and emotional space. Indeed, at the Body and Soul conference in February 1996 we heard how many elderly people in a care of the elderly ward would turn their faces to the wall when they were trying to pray, but find interruptions all the time, and basically friendly, helpful nurses asking them if they were all right. Indeed, supposing one did want quiet for prayer, or even to have an understandable little weep, it is hard to imagine how most of us would achieve that in the standard health-care setting, particularly in wards for the elderly which are all too often very overcrowded, and where staff have an inclination to infantilise their patients by constantly cheering them up and chivvying them along, when rest and peace and contemplation are what is desired.

In Christianity, sacramental ministry is often needed by the sick or dying. That has to be provided by ordained clergy in almost all cases, as it does, if genuinely sacramental, at the funeral service. Since funerals are often the best way of encouraging and helping the bereaved to 'let go', real energy and thought have to be devoted to how the funeral should best be conducted. The fact that a clergyperson has conducted hundreds of funerals in the past does not mean that he or she will get it right for this particular person, this parti-cular family, this time, and difficult decisions have to be made as to whether the funeral is for the living or the dead. It is not, after all, uncommon to find people who are dying, busily planning their own funeral. Indeed, macabre stories abound of people who are visited by hospital chaplains or, preferably, their own clergy if they are religious and have a priest or a rabbi or someone, discussing with real enthusiasm how their funeral is to be conducted, down to the choice of readings and music.

Yet I cannot help feeling that there is a real difficulty here. Though it is excellent that so many dying people become so animated in discussions about their own funerals, and though, as officiant at several funerals, I have often thought that the person who had died is somehow watching to make sure I get it right and it is just as he or she wanted it, in fact the funeral is not for the deceased but for the living. It is not up to the dying person to try to organise things beyond the grave, though one can see how being able to give instructions beyond the grave can give immense satisfaction. Yet, if the funeral is for the living and not for the dead, then it should be the bereaved who are consulted about the funeral. One thing healthcare workers can do if they spot the forthcoming funeral becoming an issue for the dying person and his or her family is to encourage them to talk about it and compromise about it, as there is clearly value in the dying person feeling that he or she is getting what he or she wants, whilst there is equally real value in the funeral being as therapeutic as it can be for the bereaved family who have to keep on living. This is no easy task, but is something that healthcare workers working with the dying, and the pastoral carers, clergy and others, all too often have to deal with.

There are several kinds of ritual. There are rites of separation, such as the bar mitzvah of a Jewish boy, or a coming of age ceremony. There are rites of transition, such as a wedding and honeymoon; rites of reincorporation or reunion, such as the dedication of a new home. A funeral service, together with the preparation beforehand which may include preparing the body for burial, and often the family gathering afterwards, has aspects of all three. There is the separation between the grieving family and the one who has died, seen in the lowering of the coffin into the grave, or symbolised by the drawing of a curtain at the crematorium. This helps the bereaved to face the reality of death, particularly where, as in a Jewish burial, the bitter memory is formed of a loud clang of a shovel full of earth landing on the coffin lid. For, unlike common Anglican practice, with a few crumbs of earth being scattered into the hole, Jews and Muslims literally bury their dead, communally. Spadefuls of earth are piled on top of the coffin. The chief mourner puts in the first spadeful, and the other mourners follow suit. There is no doubt that separation is very fully marked by what is a brutal, but useful, tradition. There is no hiding the finality as you hear the lumps of clay descend.

But the funeral also serves to remind the living to face their own eventual death. The prayers commend the loved one to God's merciful keeping, so that some of the pain of separation is handed to God. But then the mourners commit themselves to God's loving care and protection, whilst the whole congregation becomes a kind of support network. So the funeral, if properly planned and really used for its purpose, can be an important part of the grieving process. It provides a formal and ritual context in which the strong emotions of grief can be appropriately and publicly acknowledged, and in which symbolically the bereaved can be helped by the whole community.

That is vital. Other rituals act as reinforcers of the grieving process, such as the visiting of the 'place of memory', even though no-one, or very few people, believe that the deceased is actually there in any real sense. Partly in the crucially important lonely weeks immediately after the funeral, and partly, also, at significant times like the first anniversary, visiting the grave helps to focus on the passage of time, and, if done in the company of someone else, allows the expression of pastoral support when tears are particularly near the surface, and where, somehow, it is acceptable that they should be.

It is interesting to note that the lack of rituals in mourning may even contribute to an inadequate resolution of grief. In those parts of our society where religious rituals are not held to be significant (which is a growing number as church attendance declines and religious observance generally is on the wane), there is a noticeable increase in the number of counselling agencies offering help to the bereaved. This is because the kind of pastoral care that bereaved people need is not religion specific, though the different theologies make it hard for the clergy of one faith, sometimes, to provide adequate bereavement counselling to people of another. Most pastoral care is, however, practical, though it may be an expression of something more theological.

Dealing with suffering

Most of us experience suffering with great difficulty, and are neither good at dealing with it pastorally, nor at dealing with it for ourselves. Most of us find it meaningless, find the fact of suffering when we could be dead (which many regard as an endless sleep) unacceptable, which explains the move towards euthanasia, and find the fact that we are suffering being out of our control quite horrific. And people still do. The great theologian Hans Kung, a strong Roman Catholic, with his colleague Jens, in their plea for euthanasia to be legalised, tell the tale of a 12-year-old girl with terminal cancer and in considerable pain, stuck in a side ward, whom the medical staff left alone to get on with dying, because they could not bear it. Yet one cannot help think that the staff could have done more, and that euthanasia might not be the only answer. Perhaps the first requirement is to deal with the loneliness, with the emotional and spiritual needs of a dying person. They may not always need to be put out of their misery. We can see the argument for fewer interventions, for kindness, not silence, for support, not chemotherapy. But, that having been said, it does not add up to a convincing argument for euthanasia.

The hospice movement has made an enormous contribution to our thinking in this area. With the gradual removal of suffering from many terminally ill people by skilled and patient pain relief, and by the kind of holistic care which looks after the whole person rather than the pain, the cancer, alone, the hospice movement has made it clear that it is possible for most of us to die with dignity, without undue suffering. We will suffer – the grief of parting, the pain which sometimes cannot be reached, the weakening, the sorrow on our loved ones' faces. But that suffering, though there, will not be the agony of intractable pain, will not be the kind of suffering which we were expected to tolerate bravely, teeth clenched, lips bitten, so that no-one could see how near we were to tears.

The hospice has allowed us to think about the meaning of death, to face our end bravely, to contemplate our end, in a way very true to the old Christian tradition of contemplating our end. No longer do we keep the coffin in the bedroom, just to remind us. Now we can die slowly, pain-free, and think about what needs to be said, what needs to be done, how we want to end our time on earth. So it is diminished suffering. Unnecessary suffering is not acceptable in the thinking of the hospice movement and the whole, now much more widespread, palliative care movement. People should not have to suffer. It is not right.

Yet we only have to turn on television news to see people in other parts of the world suffering in their deaths, the man crawling on his hands and knees in Rwanda, in the sight of aid workers, with half his head blown off, in agony, but with the aid workers knowing they too would be shot if they went anywhere near him. That is suffering – both for the man himself and for those watching him die a slow, protracted, agonised death.

So too is watching the suffering of a small baby where anaesthesia is not working or is too strong for the tiny frame to take, or the suffering of an old person who has no physical pain, but is beginning to dement, and knows it.

There is no shortage of suffering in our world, and when we think about suffering in death, we can begin to think how fortunate we are in the western world, and particularly in Britain, with its highly skilled and supported hospice movement, that we suffer much less in death than many other people. And that we believe that suffering in death should be minimised. That belief, and the fact that pain in dying has reduced considerably with the skill of palliative care teams, has led to a diminution in fear of death, particularly amongst the elderly.

Indeed, the fear that exists tends to be more about the process of dying than of death itself, and a regret, an anger, at having to leave this world and all that is familiar in it. Yet we look at suffering people, and begin to wonder if there is not more that can be done. For instance, is the person with dementia suffering? Or is it that we suffer in advance at the thought of being demented? Or is it that we found so terrible, so distressing, our own aged parents or others who were demented, and seemed to us to live miserable lives? What is the nature of suffering here, and how do we come to terms with it?

Thinking like this will itself make us face up to what we want and do not want, indeed will make us become clearer about our own beliefs, and make us value some of those moments of intimacy in conversation more than ever. Indeed, forcing ourselves to discuss these issues, these deeper questions, requires far greater thought about suffering than occurs at present, despite our extraordinarily successful and much loved hospice movement. What we desire and do not desire as individuals is something we have rarely faced up to. If we can do it as individuals, we might even be able to do it as a society, and think about what expectations should be for most of us as we face our ends.

Religion and culture

How we die and how we are buried or cremated, how we grieve and whom we include in our grief, is coloured by different attitudes to death and dying in different cultures. People are variously affected by the religions and cultures in which they grew up, whether or not they have actually practised that particular religion or followed that way of life in the rest of their lives. Catholics who could only be described as 'lapsed' have a tendency to want last rites. Jews who have not been near a synagogue for 50 years want a Jewish burial and someone to say 'kaddish', the mourner's prayer, for them. Sikhs want the ritual readings of the Guru Granth Sahib even though they have not been near a gurdwara for years, and so on. See Chapter 5 for further information on religion and culture.

Whether it is a fear of the unknown that brings people back to their religious and cultural observances when they are dying, we will never really know. For it is confused by the fact that most people die in relative old age and there is a tendency to return to religious belief and cultural practice with age anyway. It also appears to have relatively little to do with faith as such. Certainly, Jews I have spent a great deal of time with in their last weeks and months have been quite frank about their lack of belief in a personal God. They have, nevertheless, wanted a proper Jewish funeral, and their family to sit shiva, going through the mourning ritual, for them.

On one level, none of this makes sense. But, on another, it is perfectly comprehensible. If we remove ourselves from the sort of thinking about religion that is particularly Christian, the idea that being a Christian means having made a specific act of faith, either at baptism or at confirmation, which is what is in a sense transformational, it is easier to understand this tendency to revert to the faith and customs of one's ancestors. For many other religious and cultural groups are not as 'faith' dominated as Christianity. This is not to suggest that they have no faith. Far from it. But it is to suggest that many of the customs that people go back to have more to do with community and less with actual belief. People belong to a cultural group as much as to a religious one. In many parts of the world, one is defined by how one buries one's dead and mourns them – as a Muslim, a Hindu, a Buddhist, a Zoroastrian, a Sikh. Often, the desire to die in a particular way or to be buried and mourned in a particular way is more about making one's peace with the cultural and religious group from which one comes. It is also, sometimes, to do with a reawakened faith, as a result of thinking time as one approaches one's end. But the motivation is extremely complicated, and often not really capable of being subjected to close analysis.

Religious funerals are also common because people in Britain associate ritual mourning with a religious service. (That is not necessarily the case in the Indian sub-continent, for instance.) So, even for those who never attend church, it is still thought appropriate for a priest or other religious leader to conduct proceedings at the cemetery or the crematorium. That may be partly because, as mentioned above, it is hard to devise a service which has any meaning which does not fit into a religious ritual. The British Humanist Association has done much to promote the kind of funeral service or service of remembrance which is non-religious, and has outline services which they will send to anyone who wants them. But such developments are relatively little known outside the big cities, though the funerals conducted by the British Humanist Association are often very moving occasions. We are beginning to see moves for green funerals, and for a variety of new style, non-religious funerals – including those developed by the Natural Death Society. Increasingly, people who are dying – and their families and friends – are thinking about new ways of treating the coffin, the body and the actual ceremony, and cardboard coffins, painted by the dying person and his or her friends, are now becoming relatively common, as are woodland funerals, with the final resting place being in a leafy glade rather than a cemetery.

But religious funerals of one kind or another are still the norm, and there may be more to it than custom. Clergy of all religions can often help the family in grieving, as can healthcare workers who have been close to the person who has died. In faiths other than Christianity, this might mean helping prepare the body for the funeral, assuring the dying person that he or she will be given a funeral, and preparing for the burial or cremation, in accordance with the customs and rules of the particular religious grouping. In Christianity, it is more likely to be done by the clergy in conjunction with the undertaker, and staff are more used to following the custom of that particular area and Christian belief. At the funeral service itself, the religious leader, of whatever faith, usually acts as leader of the congregation and sets the tone, both of grief and of thanksgiving for the life of the person who has died, in conjunction with the rest of the community where that is appropriate.

For there is little thinking about grief in the rituals surrounding death in much of Britain and the United States. Yet the United States has taken the art of funerals to excess. The embalmer has a field day in America, cemeteries are like theme parks, people are dressed in glorious clothes when they are put in the coffin (casket) for their funeral, there is a kind of glorying in the expense of funerals and in the way of showing love by having a bigger and better coffin with more and more luxurious linings or with better, and bigger, brass handles. People are made up to look better than they ever did in real life by the morticians' beauticians. To some of us, all this seems a bit sick. Yet it is one way of dealing with the agony death inevitably brings. (And some elements of that thinking are creeping over to this side of the Atlantic, with more questions about the kind of coffin, and the expense to be laid out, than was hitherto the case. Finally, the public is beginning to learn about the colossal cost of funerals, and the idea that one should save up for one's funeral is rapidly disappearing, with dying people telling their children to go for the cheapest option.)

The problem with it is that, when the funeral is over, when the body has been viewed in its glory, there is nothing afterwards. The money has been spent, the body buried, and the bereaved have nowhere to go, nothing to do, no automatic visitors to call on them. When Jessica Mitford wrote *The American Way of Death* and drew attention to the excesses, she did not point out the lack of a grieving process within all this. Profit for the morticians is there for the picking. Support for the bereaved is harder to find.

Yet with both the British and American Protestant traditions coming out poorly in terms of support for the bereaved in any structured way (many individual communities are very good at providing informal support), it is nevertheless from this tradition, in Britain, that the modern hospice movement sprang. Dame Cicely Saunders, OM, is a profoundly believing Christian, and her foundation, St Christopher's Hospice, is an institution with a strong Christian, slightly evangelical, feel to it. The other, older, leading hospices in London, Trinity in Clapham and St Joseph's in Hackney, also have a Christian feel to them – in the case of St Joseph's, Catholic, in the case of Trinity, High Anglican. But it was Dame Cicely who founded the modern philosophy of pain control. It was she who found the fact that people were dying in pain quite unacceptable. At least part of her revulsion was related to her Christian faith – the journey to the afterlife should be a good one, and the good death was a goal much to be desired.

There are many people who would argue that the fact that the modern hospice movement grew up in Britain is related to the proverbial British 'stiff upper lip', the sense that, whatever the pain, whatever the tragedy, we may not scream out with it. Though there may be a grain of truth in that, the root-edness in the Christian tradition is more compelling as an explanation. To journey on well into the afterlife, one should have a good death – die well, in fact. Meanwhile, for committed Christians caring for the terminally ill, there is much to be gained spiritually from helping to alleviate their pain, in order to allow them to focus on their end – and on the next life.

The hospice movement has gone far wider than Christianity now, but it has its roots inescapably in a Christian view. Apart from anything else, the medieval hospices, places to rest one's head, were Christian institutions, and part of that thinking has found its way into modern hospices. So too has much of the thinking behind the strongly Christian nursing orders in the Catholic church, the only nurses in much of the 18th and 19th centuries (until Florence Nightingale) who would provide tender care. For after the control of the nursing and midwifery guilds was taken over by the medical colleges in the 16th and 17th centuries, the noble calling of nursing became an occupation for drunken women of no great skill or character, unless it was undertaken by women of the church. So Christianity played a large part in such good nursing care that was available. Even after Florence Nightingale, and her success in getting nursing taken seriously as a profession for women of good family, there was a strongly Christian edge to it. Even in modern times, young nurses in training at St Thomas' Hospital in London were expected to pray in the wards every day.

That Christian tradition of care for the sick and dying has been very strong. Its absence from the care of those who live on is therefore all the more remarkable. Yet modern Christians are thinking more about bereavement counselling than ever they did, and there is more of an organised attempt to get visitors going to the houses of those who have been bereaved. Yet, with all that modern Christians have done for the welfare of the dying, there is a hole in their care of the living which still needs to be filled.

Social networks

There is a growing network of bereavement support agencies throughout the UK. Some are really excellent, and encourage people to talk about their loss in a way few others can. Others are less good. But, even at their least effective, they offer someone to whom the bereaved person or people can talk without fear that they will be thought to be mad, and without fear that anything they say will go any further. Whether the service offered is bereavement counselling as such, or simply the helping hand and ear of someone who has been through the same, is in a way irrelevant. What needs to be done is to make sure that someone who has been bereaved, particularly someone who does not come from a community which is clearly going to take over, is put in touch with whatever services are available. That is particularly important for those who are Anglicans, broadly speaking, or people of no particular faith. For the Anglicans, it is because their churches do not provide such a listening and supportive service, on the whole. For the others, it is because they have no church or equivalent, but still need to have a chance to grieve in a structured way.

All these are things which can help the bereaved. All of them are things where the chaplains of a hospital or hospice, grossly overworked as they often are, can provide a good deal of the training. Healthcare professionals can guide people towards such support. But this is not a matter primarily for healthcare professionals, though they have taken a surprising lead in this area within the hospice and palliative care world. This is a matter for society, and for the social networks which ordinary people have, and where isolated people need to be introduced, in order for them to gain support.

Whether a family have traditional bereavement rituals or not, the value of the social network, and the fact that people are increasingly talking about the dead person, and coming up and giving words of comfort, is much to be welcomed. It is now comparatively rare for people to cross the street when they see a bereaved person coming, because they are embarrassed and do not know what to say. Much more, even if there is no clear ritual, people will say something: 'I am sorry for your grief'. They will send a sympathy card, a growing phenomenon and much to be welcomed, and they will write a condolence letter, as they always did, and say in it that they will be in touch, and truly be in touch. All of this is much to be valued, and has changed hugely for the better. But, even then, it is as well to describe it more, encourage it more, institutionalise it more. For that kind of support through a loved one's dying and after their death is probably the best that we can do.

Recognising the spiritual and developing a sensitivity to spiritual care

For many health professionals, as with other people in our society, some of this is very hard to do. The difficulty many of us encounter in thinking and talking about grief comes from a variety of causes. First, there is our own lack of experience of death, something discussed earlier. Many health professionals will not have seen a dead person as part of their normal growing up. Granny was not laid out in the front room, but died hygienically, if not necessarily happily, in a hospital bed. In urban societies death is cleared away, is untidy and is planned not to be something for us all to deal with. Secondly, when deaths have occurred, many of us will have experienced funerals which are a pale imitation of what our grandparents will have known, whatever our religion or cultural background. There will have been little weeping or wailing, whatever the community. There will have been a relatively perfunctory service, even though, in some cultures and traditions, the mourning rituals are themselves quite rich. As children growing up, experiencing the deaths of grandparents and others, our experiences are unlikely to have been of great ceremonial or of rich funereal traditions, or even, for many of us, of fully explored mourning. It is hard, therefore, for us to empathise properly with grief. We have so little experience of it. And health professionals, often younger than their patients, will have less experience of grief than older people, on the whole.

Thirdly, the term spirituality has somehow become caught up in a whole series of ways of thinking which can be either helpful or profoundly unhelpful, but where many of us have a considerable lack of clarity about what is required to proffer any sort of spiritual (as opposed to religious) understanding. This is because of a mixture of things – new age spirituality is not necessarily the same as the sense of holiness, of a spiritual awareness, old-fashioned Christians would experience in their churches on the great holy days. That is, in its turn, different again from the type of intense spirituality to be found in some Buddhist meditation, or in the celebration of festivals in Islam, with all the bustle there might be in the mosque, leading to a kind of enriched religious fervour. Then, there is the spirituality associated with the experience of home rituals such as the sabbath evening in Jewish homes, the spirituality of glowing faces in the candlelight around the table.

This is all about spirituality. Some of it is attached to particular kinds of religious rituals, religious feelings. But the soaring of the spirit, the awareness of something other, the heightening of the emotions, the sensitivity to something above and beyond us, can occur in a variety of ways at different times. And that idea of spirituality, of the heightening of emotions and sensitivity to something above and beyond us, can be muddied by some of the sentimentality to be found in some new age thinking, or in some of the celebrations of religious festivals in almost all religions, where the point gets lost, where most is done for form, but where there is a slightly oleaginous sense of worthiness, of comfort out of the fact that other people are joining in too, which is not what spirituality is about.

Dying people often have a very heightened spiritual awareness. Some people have it when they have never experienced anything like it before in their lives, and indeed they find it one of the enriching things of the dying process. But some people loathe the feeling that they are ebbing away, and sense the spiritual nearness of 'the other' at the same time as feeling they are moving into another world, another plane. This is not to be confused with 'out of body' experiences. This is not about being out of the body. It happens as a result, some say, of drugs. Others say it comes about as a result of weakness. People who have been very weak in quite different circumstances, temporarily, often talk of the sense of heightened emotions they have, and much of what dying people talk about may be related to the heightened emotions of extreme physical weakness. Whatever the cause, the sense of this heightened spiritual awareness is pleasant for some and deeply disturbing for others, who feel as if their personalities are changing. Health professionals who are caring for people who are experiencing this heightened awareness need to be sensitive to it, need to know that it is normal, and need to understand that for some people it is hugely enriching. For, when people accept it willingly, even seek it, they find that they gain something from the process of dying beyond the settling of accounts, the talking and reconciliation that many people who die well seek to achieve. They gain an insight, an insight they often try to convey to the rest of us. It has something to do, often, with a lack of fear. It can be expressed for some in the words of Canon Henry Scott Holland: 'I am only in the next room ...', as a sense of unbelievable nearness to those whom one is leaving. It can also be something to do with an experience of Heaven. It varies from individual to individual, from cultural group to cultural group. And people will see, with that heightened awareness, different things according to their own backgrounds.

One example which springs to mind is a story about my father and a nurse who was caring for him when he had just come out of intensive care at a leading London teaching hospital. My father was a non-orthodox Jew who was brought up orthodox, and whose underlying attitudes were very typical of traditional Jewish thought. The nurse concerned was a young, religious, Irish Catholic. She had been in the same bed in intensive care as my father after an allergic reaction to a hepatitis injection some weeks earlier. As she was sitting chatting to my father, trying to keep him awake, he started telling her about what he had seen when he had woken up and found a tube down his throat. He had looked around and seen all these shadowy figures dressed in grey, and everything was dark, shadowy and silent. So he had known he was in Sheol, the pit, the place where dead people go in the earliest Hebrew Bible traditions, where everything is colourless and nothing has any real shape. The nurse looked at him quizzically and then said that she had woken up with the same experience, except that she had looked around and seen all those figures dressed in shining white, and she had looked across and there was a cross on the wall, and there was bright shining golden light every-where. She had been convinced it was Heaven until she realised her grand-mother was not there. If it were Heaven, her grandmother would definitely have been there.

When my father was a little better, she took him over to see what the inten-sive care unit was really like, what they had actually seen. The staff were dressed in green. It was painted cream and green. The imagined cross was breathing equipment on the wall. There was a great deal of noise and people talked to each other and conveyed information about how their patients were doing. This was not the grey shadowy place of Sheol nor the bright white shining place of Catholic Heaven. Yet both of them had seen what they had been conditioned, probably as quite small children, to expect to see. And both found it both funny, and deeply worrying, that their minds worked like that.

Yet the story conveys an important lesson. Spiritual awareness, a heigh-tened look at the world, may give false images of reality. It may be some-thing we expect to see, to feel. But as staff caring for people who have these experiences, our responsibility lies in understanding it, in dealing sensitively with it, in not spending our time saying something is 'not true', or that people are hallucinating. For they may indeed be hallucinating. But often something much more complicated is taking place, due to pain, and weakness, and early teaching, and a sense of being partly here, partly else-where. It should not be mocked, but people who have such experiences should be encouraged to talk to us about them, at least in part because some of them will find this whole stage of experiencing the strange deeply disturbing, and health professionals can be very reassuring: 'It is entirely normal. You are not alone'. Every person has different experiences, but the fact that they can be told that it is not unusual to go through this stage is comforting. And, for those who are getting immense pleasure, huge spiritual succour, and enrichment from this heightened awareness, it is an enormous pleasure to be able to talk about it, to recount the experience of joy and relief. But, for those of us with little religious background, and little understanding of spirituality, it is an education in itself, and we have to train ourselves to watch out for the signs of a developing spiritual sense in our patients, and be prepared to be supportive.

References

1 Social and Community Planning Research (1992) *British Social Attitudes Survey.* Social and Community Planning Research, Dartmouth.
2 Body and Soul. A first national conference at the Derbyshire Royal Infirmary in February 1996. Organised by Mark Cobb and Vanessa Robshaw. The proceedings were published in 1998. Cobb M and Robshaw V (1998) *The Spiritual Challenge of Health Care.* Churchill Livingstone, Edinburgh.

5

Religious beliefs and customs

This chapter will provide some headlines which may be useful to anyone who wishes to understand what people of other faiths experience as the meaning of the last great experience. For most of us, such knowledge helps us sympathise with those of other faiths and cultural groups when they are bereaved, and, for health professionals, there is no doubt that we care better when we know something about the traditions and beliefs of our patients, and try not to impose our own beliefs upon them, particularly in the face of death. For those who want more detailed information than what is available here, I have written a book particularly about caring for dying people of different faiths,[1] which may be helpful. There are also many other books dealing with cultural and religious differences, some of which are listed in the bibliography.

Traditionally, the three Abrahamic faiths, Judaism, Christianity and Islam, had some kind of a view of the afterlife, although it was more or less clearly defined according to which religion and also according to which bit of which religion. Eastern religions tended to have more ideas about reincarnation as some other being and constant reinvention of the self in different species. Whatever, the clear evidence is that ideas about Heaven and Hell, afterlife and so on are changing and have a less strong hold on us than once they did. Yet, the British Social Attitudes Survey suggests belief in an afterlife is still very strong in our society.[2] 55% of people in Britain believe in life after death (admittedly compared with 78% in Northern Ireland and the USA and 80% in the Irish Republic), 54% believe in Heaven (compared with 86% in the USA, 87% in the Irish Republic and 90% in Northern Ireland), and the only really low-scoring belief is in Hell, where the British show a mere 28%, compared with 71% in the USA, 53% in the Irish Republic and 74% in Northern Ireland.

Added to that, there is clear evidence from all the interviews conducted with people who have been dying and those who are bereaved that in some way they believe they will be reunited with their dear ones after death. Young and Cullen in their *A Good Death* cite the extent to which the people who had died became ghosts or spirits or manifestations of the deceased. To some extent the dead become comforting – they can be summoned at any time and can help the living to cope with their suffering in bereavement. They carry on beyond the parting. The older people, particularly, who expected to die themselves relatively soon, looked forward to joining their spouses or whoever after death, and being reunited with dear ones they had lost, often far too early. But there is an important contrast they noticed between their informants and the ones Gorer (1965) had interviewed 30 years earlier, where people had talked of not worrying about money in Heaven, or thought that in the next life there would always be sunshine and daylight. Despite Young and Cullen's (1996) sample not suggesting quite such literal things about the next life, the emphasis on reunion with those who have already died is so strong as to suggest a still present sense of the afterlife which has many of the characteristics of this life, certainly in the sense of people being distinguishable and their personalities being the same, with them remaining able to look after the ones who are still alive. And there is no doubt that people find such ideas comforting.

These are not the beliefs of people who have no sense of something to come, some afterlife, however ill-defined. After all, sometimes it is even more difficult for the human mind to come to terms with the idea of actually going nowhere. The idea that this is the end, finality, and that there is nothing more to give additional meaning to what has gone before, to what one might even feel one had wasted, is painful for most of us. The ideas of Heaven and Hell respond to a deep human need to feel that there is something after all this, whatever it may be, and there is justice in this world, or at least the next, so that the sinner gets his or her just deserts and the good person who lived in penury all his or her life, with his or her goodness unrecognised, uncelebrated, gets the glories of Heaven.

That idea is somehow very appealing. It is interesting to reflect on the fact that ancient Judaism did not have such a concept of Heaven and Hell, and that Christianity probably got it from some other religion than Judaism, maybe Mithraism. However, some rather ill thought through idea of Heaven (much less about Hell, though Gehenna is mentioned) began to appear in Jewish literature in the early Christian centuries. Clearly, the idea of getting one's just deserts in some world was catching on. The answer to 'Why do the wicked prosper?' has been found. It was that they prospered only in this world, and they met with their just deserts in the torment of the next.

Suffering

This is the age-old religious problem of the theodicy. If God is just, how can He allow the innocent to suffer, allow people to live in poverty, allow children to die painfully of acute cancers, allow the death of the destitute in earthquakes and floods? The answer, for those who take this view, lies in what happens to those people who have suffered so in the next life. They will get their reward in Heaven. Whilst the sinners who 'ground the faces of the poor' and never did anything for anybody, who lived well as others suffered, will go to Hell, and suffer eternal torment. That thinking satisfies the natural human desire for justice. It also satisfies the desire to have a God who is just, who allows human suffering in order to test people (in Judaism these are called the sufferings of love), and will reward the good and punish the evil in the next life. It even allows us to enjoy revenge – a revenge, described as punishment, executed by God, and not part of what human beings feel as the desire to execute revenge themselves.

But for any of this system of reward and punishment to mean anything, people have to be aware of death all the time. So Christianity reminds its adherents that 'In the midst of life we are in death'. Other religions remind us that we must die. Few religions allow us to carry on in bemused and attractive innocence, for if we do, we will not take the reward and punishment system seriously. We are not allowed to forget. (Other faiths have similar ways of doing things, which will be dealt with below.) Somehow, this reward and punishment system is supposed to make us feel that being ill, suffering, is part of the divine plan, is our way of earning our way into heaven.

Christianity

History

Christianity is the religion of the followers of Jesus, whom they proclaimed to be the Son of God and through whom they approached God himself. The extent to which Jesus is viewed as part of the godhead varies according to which branch of Christianity is under consideration. Most tenets of the faith are the same, whichever group is being examined, but the emphasis sometimes varies, as for instance with the concept of the virgin birth: some sections of Christianity are emphatic about it, while others are less dogmatic about its literal truth.

The fundamental belief of Christianity dates back to Jesus, born in Bethlehem some 2000 years ago. He was born into a Jewish family and community and fitted into a school of charismatic teaching and miracle working of contemporary Galilee. He taught and performed his miracles mainly during the last three years of his life, in areas which are now part of now modern Israel, Jordan and Syria. The country was then under Roman rule, under the governor Pontius Pilate.

His followers believed Jesus to be the Messiah, the anointed one, saviour of the Jews. The word in Greek for Messiah is Christos, meaning anointed one, hence the name Christ and Christian. Jesus was an extremely successful and charismatic figure, and attracted a large following. In itself, that inspired jealousy in some, who felt threatened by his popularity. They, along with the Roman rulers of the time, wanted to overthrow him and so, in approximately 33 AD, Jesus was crucified just outside Jerusalem. According to the New Testament, he was buried, rose again on the third day, and is the saviour of the world, and the symbol of sacrifice for human sins.

Specific beliefs and customs

A proper discussion of what death means in theological terms is rapidly disappearing from almost all faiths. Christianity has a framework within which dying and grieving can be faced. It affirms that God offers grace sufficient to help Christians to cope. Earlier generations of Christians made much more of 'preparing for a good death' than many would nowadays. In the rubric for 'The Visitation of the Sick' it says:

> *Then shall the Minister examine whether he repent him truly of his sins, and be in charity with all the world; exhorting him to forgive, from the bottom of his heart, all persons who have offended him; and if he hath offended any other, to ask them forgiveness; and where he hath done injury or wrong to any man, that he make amends to the uttermost of his power. And if he hath not before disposed of his goods, let him then be admonished to make his Will, and to declare his debts, what he oweth and what is owing to him; for the better discharging of his conscience, and the quietness of his Executors. But men should often be put in remembrance to take order for the setting of their temporal estates whilst they are in health. (Book of Common Prayer, 1662)*

It is not hard to see that the attitude in that period (and for some believing Christians to this day) is that people should prepare for death. Contemplating one's death is something a Christian is instructed to do. Earlier generations lived in constant fear and awareness of death, and would keep a coffin open beside the bed. Others would confess their sins before they went to sleep every night, in case they should not wake up. The fear of going to sleep and dying in the night was one which Victorian children were taught to experience. We had to be afraid of death, because if we had lived a wicked, unrepentant life in this life, we would go to Hell. The importance of ideas about Heaven and Hell is critical. Most modern Christians in Britain would argue that Heaven and Hell are to be taken figuratively rather than literally, yet there is still a horror of what happens after death if one is not to go to Heaven, but to some as yet unspecified (since traditional Hell is out of fashion) torment, including, in some people's views, the Hell of not being remembered at all, or only being remembered for evil, and not for good.

It seems to me that the Christian idea of the afterlife, however liberally interpreted, means a form of Heaven, of eternal bliss, which comes about as a result of the relationship with Jesus. People who do badly in this life, or who fail to take Jesus into their lives in some way, to follow his teachings, are doomed, by some Christians at least, to Hell and eternal torment. For most Christians, Heaven and Hell are concepts rather than literal truth, but the central theme of the theology is that of a new spiritual birth taking place as a result of putting Jesus at the centre of one's existence. Therefore, terminally ill Christians may seek to put Jesus at the centre of the end of their lives, and there is a well attested phenomenon of irreligious people who were brought up Christians, especially Catholics, seeking to return to their faith and to Jesus at the end of life.

In Christianity, death is an evil used by God as a sign of his judgement on anything ungodly about life. It is threatened for those who take no notice of God's will. But the paradox, as well as the climax, of the Gospels is that Jesus himself dies. Jesus, God incarnate, suffers death as the judgement of God. That shows both that death is universal, though it is rarely interpreted that way by Christians, and that those who hold good Christian faith in Jesus will somehow be saved, although they will actually, physically, die. Jesus's death was one of pain and torment. Yet, according to Christian theology, Jesus atoned for the sins of humanity through his death, so that, providing human beings are willing to accept him, and recognise his atonement, they will be saved and freed from an end in torment during and after death. So baptism gives grace, and confirmation affirms belief. For the Christian, the 'sting' of death is given relief.

Yet, though that is very satisfactory in theory, it does not always help the dying person who was brought up a Christian. For, facing their own mortality, they are still afraid, rightly so, as many would say. They do not find the death of Jesus helpful, though some find the idea of God raising him from the dead more comfortable, though they are not convinced that everyone is to be given that kind of resurrection. Nevertheless, there is hope of resurrection for Christians who meet their maker at their death. For believing Christians, that can be very comforting, and enormously rewarding as a way of thinking about death, and its meaning. For Jesus is perceived as a 'sure and certain hope' of human resurrection, and that hope should help Christians to face their deaths as a gift of divine love, leading as it does, according to this way of thinking, to resurrection. But it is not always so, for many Christians are not so certain about resurrection, or indeed about the veracity of the story of the Cross. As historical criticism bites at many Christians' thinking about the Gospel stories, as some modern theologians take an increasingly symbolic, interpretative view of the synoptic gospels, then it becomes more difficult for many Christians to take much of the theology literally, because they have partially rejected the story as in the Gospels. That very rejection of historical veracity makes them also lose a sense of certainty about what they will find after death. Theological uncertainty, as a result of historical doubts or new knowledge, breeds a kind of loss of equanimity in the face of death, which is arguably the great theological and emotional test for us all.

Yet Christianity, more than other faiths perhaps, has made the process of grief, the idea of pain, part of a way of ennobling the spirit. Unlike many other religions, Christianity believes suffering can be, and often is, good for people. Theologians talk of the pain that heals, of suffering bringing one to a deeper level, or higher level, of existence. There are similar ideas in Buddhism, but the theology of Christianity is one that adulates suffering, in a very particular way, and therefore might have been expected to make more, in a ritualised way, of the grieving process. Since suffering can be seen, at least in some regards, as a way into a process of sharing in the redemptive sufferings of God in Jesus, one might have expected there to be more attempt to make that a concrete part of the grieving process, ritualised to make its significance clear. Then suffering can be the route to comfort and transformation, which, in a sense, is part of the Christian message. But, curiously, it is not there in the grieving process after a death.

Last rites and funeral customs

It is also worth knowing something about the last rites customs of different Christian groups, because the assumption is often made that one will understand when it is quite possible that one had not realised that there were major differences. Central to these differences are the relying on 'last rites' especially for Catholics and orthodox Christians, with a final confession, being anointed with the oil of the sick, and taking communion for the last time. This can be hard when a person is really no longer able to swallow, and finds communion almost impossible to take. Nurses are often very skilled at helping someone to place a wafer on the tongue, or a drop of wine on the lips, even when it is difficult to get it swallowed, and many dying people find it very comforting to taste the wine if no more. Chaplains in hospitals and hospices are well-used to this, but sometimes when people are dying at home and have had no contact with a priest or clergyman, there are real difficulties in making the contact and allowing someone to rediscover, or even discover, their Christian faith and go through some kind of last rites within the space of a few hours. For that reason, people who are not necessarily involved in the church, but wish to support people who are terminally ill, and help them to die at ease with themselves, might need to know just enough to be able to help comfort the individual, help them (where appropriate) have some form of last rites, and sit with them until a priest or clergyman can be found.

It is also worth knowing, at an earlier stage, whether someone is either a Jehovah's Witness, who will not use blood products at any point in care, including a life-saving blood transfusion if it were needed, or a Christian Scientist, who will not allow any conventional treatment at all. Most Jehovah's Witnesses and Christian Scientists will make their position very clear at the point of entering any hospice or hospital, or to any community healthcare facility. But, occasionally, people's long abandoned beliefs come back at the end of their lives, and hospice staff recount occasional brushes with people who had been brought up as Jehovah's Witnesses, long abandoned their belief, but – at the end of their life – decided to refuse a transfusion which would not have cured them or done anything long term, but would have enhanced the quality of their lives for a few weeks or months. Jehovah's Witnesses are a relatively small group in the UK, who have been persecuted considerably in other places, but they, Plymouth Brethren, Seventh Day Adventists and Christian Scientists, are all small Christian minorities whose needs will be different from the mainstream.

Yet Christianity, particularly as practised in England in the Church of England rite, has lost many of its grieving rituals. Indeed, there are those who think that people should be positively encouraged to ritualise some of the grieving process, to force them to work through some of the stages of their grief through ritual. The Church of England has been less than active in promoting this view, partly because of its own lack of rituals, than it might have been. Christianity in Ireland, however, both north and south, both Catholic and Protestant, shows a high regard for the rituals surrounding a death, with the respect paid to 'the removal' of the body by the undertaker and the mass attendance, as a communal duty, at any funeral. Everyone goes to a funeral, to support those who are bereaved, and everyone also goes to drink and eat afterwards, at the 'wake' (watch) in order to show support to the family, and to play a part in communal grieving. It is an important part of ordinary life.

The contrast with the standard middle-class Church of England funeral in England could not be more extreme. Though the service may be very beautiful in both cases, and may even be using an identical liturgy, it is what happens afterwards that is so different. In England, the likelihood is that the mourners will go back to the house for a glass of sherry and a curling up sandwich. Or there may not even be that. There will be no prayers at the house, no regular system of callers coming for the first few days. The standard practice of people crossing the street away from someone who has just been bereaved continues, not because they wish to be unkind, but because there is not a standard, ritualised way of greeting the bereaved, a standard way of saying what one has to say – 'I am sorry. Can I do anything for you?' – in such a way that it is a standard greeting to the newly bereaved. And so the bereaved are isolated, whilst in other Christian societies the expectation would be that the entire community would come to pay its last respects to the departed.

The growth of the black churches in the UK has led the way in teaching other Christians, in England particularly, how to grieve. Many of the black churches, whether Pentecostalist or others, will treat the funeral as a mixture of a truly joyful occasion, celebrating the journey of the dead person to Heaven, and an occasion for public, emotional outpourings, including wailing and tears. The atmosphere at a funeral in one of these churches could not be more different from that in a standard Church of England church, and there is no doubt that many black Christians of West Indian origin find the standard Church of England variety of funeral cold – and insufficient to pay credit to the dead or ensure them on their way to Heaven. Black African funerals also have an element of this joy and intensity – they also often have more of the deliberate wailing and structured demonstration of grief, as well as some evocation of a spirit world (in some cases) and a concern that the dead person's body should not have the chance to be entered or taken over by spirits, so it is never left alone. In all Afro-Caribbean traditions, everyone in a community goes to the funeral – they have to be there, for the dead person's sake, for their own sake, and for the community. It is a communal activity to bury or cremate the dead.

That action of going to the funeral, or the wake, in Ireland or in much of rural Scotland, is not only about paying one's respects to the dead. One does not even have to have liked the person concerned. The wake is for the living. It is for the living that one goes to the funeral, for the living that one goes to the wake and talks about the dead person. It is an important part of community life, of good neighbourliness, to go to the wake. In most cases, a fair amount of alcohol will be consumed. But there are 'dry' wakes, where there is a strong view against alcohol. Even sitting drinking tea, and eating vast quantities of fruit cake, talking about the dead person, there is a strong sense of bonding of the community with the bereaved, and a way of ritualising the saying of farewells, and giving of comfort, to make it easier for everyone to know what to do.

Particularly in Britain, where Christianity, despite being little practised, is the official religion, it is less a question of going back to community, and more a question of sorting out what one believes theologically, that is required.

Other societies have other ways of doing it. In China, Chinese Christians have mourning customs not unlike their Chinese neighbours. In India, Indian Christians have similar customs to their Indian neighbours, Hindu, Muslim or Sikh. In Italy, people mourn in traditional ways and there are special foods. Similarly in Greece, where there are also, in some parts, old folk rituals that almost certainly predate Christianity. Each country has its mourning rituals, as does each faith. But what has happened to much of Christianity in Britain and in the United States is perhaps the result of, or a curious effect of, the puritanical view of some of Protestantism. Emotions were buttoned up. One did not speak about them. The old rituals of prayers on the third, sixth and ninth days after a death disappeared, often in a flurry of anti-Catholic feeling. So grieving became an entirely personal process, without much community help. And, as a result, though that Puritanism no longer exists, much of the Protestant approach (and Catholic in those societies as well) has lost any sense of communal involvement in grieving, in helping people to mourn.

Hints for healthcare professionals

Guilt at having 'lapsed' from Christian practice of whatever kind has to be handled with care. Emotions range from fear to devotion, to guilt at having 'lapsed', to expectation of a wonderful afterlife. The emotions are very mixed, and it is hard for those of a different faith, as it is with people of any faith group, to explore these ideas in detail. It is often helpful to call in a sympathetic priest or even lay visitor who has some understanding of Christian theology as well as the psychological effects of terminal illness and grief. At the same time, if somebody like this is not available, it can be helpful to allow the person who is dying to spill out some of his or her concerns. But pastoral visits from clergy and others can be very helpful indeed to Christians, for, more than adherents of other faiths, however 'lapsed', it tends to be theological questions they wish to address. That, combined with the need for last rites for some Christians groups, is the main reason to take particular care of the spiritual needs of Christians.

Islam

Islam is one of the world's fastest growing religions. There are Muslims in almost all countries, and Europe, hitherto thought to have a small Muslim population, has over 30 million Muslims, excluding those in Turkey, with something around one million in Britain. Most Muslims in Britain have their origins in the Indian sub-continent, but significant groups of Muslims in Britain originate from Turkey, Cyprus, Malaysia, and all over the Middle East, as well as a growing number of people who come originally from different traditions who have converted to Islam. There is also a growing number of Muslim communities in Britain whose journey to the UK has been that of persecution and terror – amongst present day asylum seekers and refugees, Muslims of a variety of kinds are the largest single faith group, coming from Bosnia, Somalia, Ethiopia, China, Kosovo, and parts of eastern Europe, to name but a few. Although not all of these people will end up staying in the UK, a sufficiently large proportion will do so for us to understand their customs and also realise that, for those who have been refugees, facing death and its attendant insecurities can make coping even more difficult.

Those Muslims whose families originated from the Indian sub-continent often have some customs that are similar to those of Hindus and Sikhs, although there are ways in which members of different faiths and traditions make themselves out as being very different from the others amongst whom they live. But those similarities between Muslim practices and Sikh and Hindu practices where families originate from the Indian sub-continent are in fact superficial. For Islam is closely related to Judaism and Christianity, and Muslim rulers have traditionally recognised members of the other two faiths as being 'people of the Book'.

History

The first tenet of Islam is that it was revealed by God (Allah) to the prophet Muhammad in Mecca, in what is now Saudi Arabia. Hence the desire on the part of many Muslims to make the pilgrimage to Mecca, the Hajj. Muhammad was born in 570 AD, leaving Mecca with his followers in 622 to escape persecution. They went to nearby Medina, where they established the true meaning of Muhammad's message. Islam became a formal, distinctive religion with its own system of government, law and rules shortly thereafter.

The beginning of the Muslim era, the way in which Muslims calculate their calendar, is from the date of the journey to Medina, entitled the Hijra. The first year is entitled 1 AH, after the Hijra. Muhammad died in 11 AH in Medina, by which time Islam had spread throughout Arabia. Islam reached India early in the eighth century, but the real Muslim influx into the Indian sub-continent was when Muslim rulers established their rule in the Punjab in the 11th century, and the Mughal dynasty from central Asia, strongly Islamic, established its rule over all of northern and central India in the 16th century with their capital in Delhi. Although Mughal power diminished by the end of the 17th century, Muslims were still a large part of the population, and when talk of independence began in the 20th century, many Muslims felt they would be overrun by the Hindu majority. So in 1947, with Indian independence, there was also partition, with the boundaries redrawn to allow a separate state of Pakistan. Indeed, there was East and West Pakistan originally, before East Pakistan broke away to become another separate Muslim state, Bangladesh. The legacy of all that unrest has not yet died away completely. There are still resentments along the Pakistani border, and great difficulties in Kashmir. Meanwhile, there are now nearly as many Muslims actually in India as in Pakistan. Yet memories of violence between Hindus and Sikhs on the one hand, against Muslims on the other, are still very present, and there are difficulties in many cases where an elderly Muslim from the Indian sub-continent is to be looked after by a Hindu, or vice versa. These things are improving, yet it is as well to be aware of sensitivities in that area.

There are two main branches of Islam, of which Sunni are some 90% and Shi'a approximately 10%. Death, martyrdom and suffering are more distinctive elements of Shi'a thought than Sunni, and it is largely (but by no means only) in Shi'a groups that the new militant Islam has its roots. As well as Sunni and Shi'a, there are also Ahmaddiya, who many Muslims do not accept as proper Muslims at all, and Ismaili Muslims, led by their prince, the Aga Khan. Ahmaddiya and Ismailis each have considerable presence in the UK, as well as Sunni and Shi'ite Muslims.

Specific beliefs and customs

The faith could be described as militantly monotheistic ('I bear witness that there is no god but Allah and Muhammad is his prophet') and although it regards Moses and Jesus as important messengers, leaders and prophets, Muhammad is the final and true interpreter.

All Muslims accept the truth of the teaching of the Holy Koran (Qur'an) and accept the code of behaviour written within it and in the recorded sayings and deeds of Muhammad. The ritual requirements of Islam, that is, the five main religious duties which very ill Muslims will wish to carry out, are faith, prayer, alms-giving, fasting and the pilgrimage to Mecca. Muslims who are terminally ill but believe that they have a little time left often still wish to make the gruelling pilgrimage to Mecca, to carry out one of the main religious obligations and therefore to die satisfied that all that can be done has been done.

Most British Muslims, but not all, especially some of the younger ones, are fairly strict about Muslim law. There is little in the way of a liberal wing of Islam in Britain, though Ismailis are often seen as the most liberal, apart from the Ahmaddiya, whom many others Muslims do not regard as proper Muslims at all. The fact that so many Muslims are fairly strict about Muslim law and traditional Islamic attitudes to many things means that those who come into contact with Muslims who are terminally ill or bereaved have a particular obligation to watch out in order not to cause offence. The requirement therefore is to know at least a little about Islam and what might be expected, and it is also always welcomed if those who are not Muslims ask in a genuinely interested way about what Muslims believe about certain things, or about Muslim customs.

There is also an increasingly important group, particularly amongst younger Muslims, of what are described as 'militant' Muslims, many of whom feel marginalised and threatened by the western world, and who want to live a completely 'Islamic' life, with no western standards and attitudes impinging. This is in part a reaction to the generally increased suspicion of young Muslims, particularly since the atrocities of 11 September 2001 – attacks carried out by al-Qaeda, but supported by many who are not directly members of that network. Young Muslims are also, separately, aware of increasing Islamophobia, a dislike, distrust and fear of Muslims which has been growing in the west for some 20 years or so.[3] These feelings of being marginalised and disliked have a powerful effect (in some cases) on how Muslims wish to be treated at the end of their lives, and, even, more importantly, how they wish their parents (whose attitudes may be very different) to be treated when facing a mortal illness. Young militant Muslims may wish for everything to be done the Muslim way, and reject much of western medicine and western attitudes. Their parents may wish to take advantage of all that western medicine has to offer, and be far less inclined to insist on the strictest of Muslim practices. This can cause tension, at the very least.

Jerusalem, Medina and Mecca are all holy cities for Muslims, because of links with Muhammad or Abraham (Muslims refer frequently to Judaism, Christianity and Islam as the three great Abrahamic faiths), but Mecca is the most sacred and important. But because the patriarchs of Judaism (Abraham, Isaac and Jacob, Moses, David, Jesus and John the Baptist, amongst others), are all thought to be fore-runners of Muhammad, the other cities are of significance. Nevertheless, Muhammad is the one to whom almost everything is referred for example. He was an 'ordinary man', frequently so described, and is not thought in any way to be a mediator between human beings and Allah, God. His teaching was that all men and women were called to Allah's service, and that they should try to live perfectly, following the Koran.

The religious duties of a Muslim are based on the so-called 'five pillars' of Islam. They are:

- faith in Allah
- daily prayer
- fasting during Ramadan
- giving alms
- making a pilgrimage to Mecca.

Prayers are always said facing Mecca, and the goal of the Hajj (pilgrimage) is always Mecca in the first instance. Every Muslim says prayers five times a day at set times, after dawn, at noon, mid-afternoon, just after sunset and at night. In Britain, with the variation of daylight hours, prayer times vary, something caring staff need to be very aware of. So the earliest prayer could be as early as three in the morning in mid-summer, whilst the last prayers could be around 11 p.m. In contrast, in winter time, prayer times run very close together.

Before prayer, Muslims wash. They stand on clean ground, or on a mat (small carpets, very often), with shoes removed and heads covered. They move in specific ways at different stages of prayer. It is worth caring staff ensuring that a devout Muslim can pray quietly, facing Mecca, and that room is given for the privacy required for a prayer mat to be kept. In winter, it may be as well to keep it out all the time, given the frequency of prayer.

It is also important to be aware of the sensitivities about modesty which is a key characteristic of all religions from the east, but which Islam takes very seriously, and which will be felt particularly strongly by the more militant younger Muslims, though it is almost universally held by Muslims in general as being very important.

How important ritual becomes often escapes those of us who are caring for people who are dying. Although we are often aware that people like to see a priest (if Catholic) and receive last rites *in extremis*, the parallels to that in other faiths often pass us by. We expect somehow the relevant chaplain (be it a rabbi, an imam, a Buddhist sister) to come by and take care of all the necessary. But in most other faiths, it does not work like this. The individual is responsible for his or her prayer. There is less in the way of sacrament, if anything at all. What needs to be done is to make it as easy as possible for the person concerned to carry out such rituals as he or she wishes to perform, without any sense that anything they wish to do is peculiar. So if a Muslim wants to be washed, or helped to wash, five times a day for prayer, that should be as ordinary as taking blood pressure. That washing requires privacy, for the face, ears, forehead, feet, hands, arms to the elbow, all need to be washed in running water, whilst some water needs to be sniffed up the nose. To add to that, a Muslim cannot pray unless, after urinating or defecation, his or her private parts have been washed in running water. A full wash in running water is also required for women at the end of a period, and for men after a nocturnal emission, whilst both sexes have to wash after sexual intercourse.

If a Muslim patient in a wheelchair needs a compass to try to discover exactly whether or not he is facing Mecca, that should not raise an eyebrow. Those rituals, the ability to carry on, to make one's peace with God in many cases, are very important, as important to a Muslim as last rites to a Catholic.

The period just before Ramadan, the major month-long fast which moves around the year because Islam sticks to the lunar calendar, is used as a time for settling disputes and ill feeling, so that for the terminally ill it can be of special significance as a last chance to solve the problems of this life, with people in this life, whoever they might be. Even if the terminally ill person does not fast, he or she may wish to make donations to charity in lieu of fasting. For Muslim law does not require the sick to fast or to observe all the normal religious laws. Indeed, Muslim law requires doing almost anything to save life – and argues that sick people should have everything possible to allow them to recover, and should in no way risk their well-being for the sake of fasting. But many terminally ill Muslims will view the particular Ramadan concerned as their last chance to observe Ramadan, and will want to do it, even though the law does not require it.

Almost all Muslims observe the dietary laws, at least to some extent. They eat no pork or pig products, and only eat 'halal' meat, slaughtered according to Muslim law, so that often, in a hospice or other hospital situation, they will only eat vegetarian food unless halal meat can be provided. Fish is permissible except for those with no fins and scales, with the exception of prawns, which are permitted. Alcohol is expressly forbidden, which can cause problems with some drug cocktails. Given the propensity these days, for hospices particularly, to offer a cocktail to patients around early evening, the fact that Muslims do not drink alcohol must be remembered and acted upon, with the exception of the more relaxed Muslims who have abandoned that prohibition.

All food to be eaten by observant Muslims has to be cooked and served separately, hence there is often an unwillingness to eat food cooked in a hospital kitchen, unless the kitchen is used to providing meals specially for Muslim patients. It is vital for caring staff to watch for this. May elderly Muslims, particularly those from the Indian sub-continent whose English is not all that good, will appear not to want to eat at all, when in fact they are worried about how the food is prepared and whether it is, according to their law, fit to eat. It is vital that caring staff watch out for elderly Muslims, especially women, apparently fading away because they do not want to eat, when not wanting to eat may be nothing at all to do with fading hunger, but because of concern about food preparation.

Last rites and funeral customs

Devout and pious Muslims believe that death is a part of Allah's plan and that to struggle against it is wrong. There is a time for death and the Koran makes that plain. Allah takes people during sleep (temporarily) and permanently when they die, at a time that is ordained. 'Allah takes the souls at the time of their death, and that which has not died in its sleep; He withholds that against which He had decreed death, but loses the other till a stated term.' (Koran, sura 39:42) Death is a necessary loss in this life, leading to the world to come. In this, as in other aspects of the faith, God's mercy is ever present: 'He has laid no hardship upon you in religion'. (Sura 22, The Pilgrimage: 78)[3] There are mystical schools, such as Ibn al-Arif, (12th Century Muslim Spain), who describe death as 'a draught of pure water to the thirsty'. For many doctors and nurses reared in the western tradition, such fatalism is very disturbing. Yet the acceptance of terminal illness, and the desire to use it as a time of surrendering to the will of Allah, means that the Muslim patient will often want less in the way of pain relief and more in the way of opportunity for prayer and contemplation. This is not to suggest that Muslims will reject pain relief (there is a strong anti-pain tradition within the religion) but Muslims will often accept less treatment for pain and its associated discomforts in order to keep awake, and use the time for seeing family and going through a time of spiritual surrendering.

Muslims believe one must accept the will of God, finally letting the dying person go, and that, whatever happens, God is good. There is spiritual growth through the experience of a cycle of a year of grief, and there is the comfort brought by the fact that the community comes to support the bereaved when all seems black and miserable.

But, before the death, there is also the fact that members of the family, and of the community, come to pray by the bed. They state the standard statement of faith first: 'There is no god but Allah, and Muhammad is his prophet', before carrying on with other prayers. That statement of faith is also supposed to be the last words a Muslim should say before he or she dies, and the desired position of a dying Muslim is with the face turned towards Mecca, whilst another Muslim whispers the call to prayer into his ear. For caring staff, this may all seem very unusual, and there will often seem to be a lot of people about watching a Muslim person die. But the family and community support is regarded as very valuable within Muslim communities, and should be encouraged and welcomed by caring staff. Indeed, they can often add to the feeling of general support for the family by making family and community members particularly welcome and by asking a very few questions about what is going on, to make it clear that it is regarded, not as mumbo-jumbo, but as an important religious ritual.

Rituals about the body are similar to those in Judaism and eastern orthodox Christianity. Most Muslims require that only other Muslims touch the body. If it is necessary for non-Muslims to do so, they should wear rubber gloves, straighten the limbs, turn the head towards the right shoulder (so that the body may be buried with the face turned towards Mecca), and wrap the unwashed body in a plain sheet. When Muslims perform these rituals for their own people, they usually straighten the body with the eyes closed, the feet tied together with a thread around the toes, and the face bandaged to keep the mouth closed. The body is usually washed by the family, at home or at the mosque, and camphor is frequently put under the armpits and into the orifices. The body is clothed in clean white cotton garments and the arms placed across the chest. Those who have been to Mecca may have brought themselves back a white cotton shroud.

Muslims are always buried, never cremated, and this is carried out as soon as possible. It can be a source of considerable distress to a terminally ill Muslim to find that there may need to be a post-mortem after a death, because of the requirement for instant burial. The body is usually taken to the graveside for prayers (though sometimes to the mosque instead) and then buried. Traditionally, Muslims would not have been buried in a coffin. But in Britain burial in a coffin is a requirement, so very plain unadorned coffins are provided. The grave also has to be marked in British law, whilst Islam would normally expect an unmarked grave. Increasingly, there are separate areas in municipal cemeteries for Muslims, which makes it all a bit easier. But where that is not the case, Muslim families can get very upset at having to bury their beloved dear departed in a burial plot next to Christians and others.

Mourning lasts around a month, whilst relatives and friends visit, bringing gifts of food, and providing support. The conversation is supposed to be about the person who has died, particularly saying good things about his or her virtues, and ignoring his or her faults. The immediate family stays at home for three days after the funeral usually, and the grave is visited on Fridays for the first 40 days, with alms being distributed to the poor. A widow should, according to Muslim law, modify her behaviour for 130 days, staying at home as much as possible, wearing plain clothes and no jewellery, presumably originally to establish whether she was pregnant or not by the deceased husband before there was any question of her remarrying.

But after the mourning procedures, the family tries to go back to normal, and the grave is rarely visited. Islam is very much this-life-affirming, so morbid obsession is uncommon. Nevertheless, the rituals of visiting and bringing food and praying over the dying person require a considerable amount of devotion from other community members, which can be a source of great comfort to the chief mourners at the time.

Hints for healthcare professionals

Those of us caring for Muslim patients who are dying, or supporting their families, should be well aware that, whatever our personal views about modesty, and particularly seeing women wearing the hijab, the veil and face covering that allows sometimes only the eyes to be seen, that these are cherished customs and that this is not the time to argue. When we are caring for others, whatever our views, and however much we might campaign for Muslim girls to be allowed to be given choices, we must respect the customs of the individuals concerned and allow them to meet their end without all their values being challenged by us.

I argue this strongly because it is very difficult. Western people, and health professionals amongst them have picked up western values more than many other groups, believe passionately in the equality of the sexes and in free choice of the individual. Often, they find themselves in a situation where the individual or the family for whom they are caring has a very different value system. Many Muslims would not cite freedom of choice as a fundamental value. They would be more inclined to rate modesty, and being at peace with God. Much of what they say might seem to less than religious westerners to be fatalistic, or at least simplistically pious. Yet it is not our role to reason or argue. In this caring mode, with people with very different views, our role is to accept, support, help and understand. In order to do that, we both need to know what we can about Islam and different Muslim customs, and to be prepared to ask.

Judaism

In some ways, it is more complicated to talk about Jews than about Muslims, despite considerable similarities, partly because the history of the Jewish people, having lived in exile amongst other people over such a long period, means that they have adopted many customs and habits of the people amongst whom they have lived.

History

Jews are a very small group in terms of world religions (an estimated 13 million), with some 400 000 Jews in the UK. Large numbers of Jews everywhere regard themselves as Jewish by peoplehood rather than by religion; nevertheless, they may well want Jewish rituals at their deathbeds, and may well want to discuss attitudes to life and death with those who are caring for them.

Judaism is the religion that developed from the religion of the ancient Israelites, as recorded in the Hebrew Bible (Old Testament). The laws of modern Judaism were established initially in about 200 CE (AD) in the Mishnah, the first codification of Jewish law, and then debated and reaffirmed in the Talmud (around 500 CE). Laws continued to be codified, and there are major differences in practice between Jews of European origin (Germany, Poland, Russia, eastern Europe) commonly referred to as Ashkenazi, from the old Hebrew word for Germany, and those from eastern and north African origins, such as Iraqi, Spanish, Portuguese, Moroccan and Algerian. The bulk of Jews in Britain are of Ashkenazi background, having arrived in Britain largely around the end of the 19th and beginning of the 20th centuries from the Polish and Russian communities, but the earliest Jews who came back in the resettlement of the Jews under Cromwell (they had been expelled from England in 1290) were Sephardi Jews who made their way from Holland, where they had lived after their expulsion from Spain and Portugal in 1492.

Judaism has developed over the centuries, and is not a completely static religion, even though orthodox Jews (the majority, by synagogue membership, but not by action, in Britain) argue that the whole of the law was given as a single entity by God to Moses on Mount Sinai, including the legal codes of the Mishnah and Talmud, as 'oral law'.

One of the great debates in the Jewish community is over the authority of the law, but the most recent history of the Jewish communities has been one of great mourning for the millions of Jews who perished under Nazi rule in the death camps of eastern Europe, and then the establishment of the State of Israel, the Jewish State.

Jews have been in Britain since 1656, though the community swelled massively from 1881–1905. Many have no connection with any synagogue, and indeed, the most recent survey of the Jewish community in Britain suggested that intermarriage between Jew and non-Jew was coming up to 50% of the community, with something under 50% being synagogue members, and indeed expressing their Jewishness in the traditional ways. This does not, however, mean that they are not expressing their Judaism in some way, though it may be more culturally than religiously. That would, however, affect the way they choose to die and be buried.

Specific beliefs and customs

The life-affirming strand in Judaism is very strong, even amongst those who are disaffected from the religion itself, and therefore a fight against death, a desire to survive no matter what, and an unwillingness on the part of many Jewish doctors to admit to their patients that they are dying, are all common features of coping with terminal illness in the Jewish community. The complications that lead on from all this for palliative care are obvious. Although honesty is a prerequisite for enabling people to cope with pain and its consequences, there are still Jewish doctors, and rabbis, and other community leaders, who feel that a Jew who knows that he is going to die will give up hope, so that his life will thereby be shortened. The strength of feeling for life in Judaism is so great that even to lose a few minutes of it is thought to be a terrible thing; indeed, all laws except three, the prohibitions against murder, idolatry and incest, may be broken to save a human life or a few minutes of it.

The result of this adulation of life is a respect for physicians within the Jewish tradition that does not always accord well with the modern view of healthcare professionals as advisers, rather than paternalistic people who tell us what to do. Life is God's gift, and the emphasis is quite clear that we had better value it, and do anything we possibly can to preserve it. Hence, doctors, physicians, are held in the highest regard because they are thought to have been given the power to heal by God. In the Talmud, at the end of the fifth century CE, we read: 'The school of Rabbi Ishmael taught: And the words: "And he shall cause him to be thoroughly healed…" (Ex. 21:19) are the words from which it can be derived that authority was given by God to the medical man to heal' (Berachot 60a). And in Ecclesiasticus (Ben Sira 38:1–2) we find: 'Honour a physician according to thy need of him, with the honours due unto him. For verily the Lord hath created him'.

So the doctor is able to cure (one hopes) and to preserve life. In this line of thought, he becomes a divine creature beyond the ordinary, because through him life can be preserved. And in the Jewish tradition, we do everything, put ourselves through everything, in order to save life, including interventions with a very small chance of success. In the commentary to the legal code, the Shulchan Aruch, we read: 'It is forbidden to cause the dying to pass away quickly; for instance, if a person is dying over a long time and cannot depart, it is forbidden to remove the pillow or cushion from underneath him'. We do not make the going easy.

Indeed, various traditional practices have been used, particularly in the medieval period, but still to be found in modern times, to avert the dread decree of death. Among them is the changing of the person's name, something that those who are concerned with the psychological welfare of the dying person should appreciate. It is thought that changing one's name averts death, since God makes up the Book of Life at every High Holy Days (the Jewish New Year, culminating 10 days later in the Day of Atonement, Yom Kippur). Those whose names are written in the Book of Life will survive for another year. Those whose names are absent will die in the course of the coming year, unless, during the 10 days between New Year and the Day of Atonement, they can avert the dread decree by good actions and putting things right between man and man and God and man.

Although relatively few modern Jews believe this is a way of deciding who is to live and who is to die, it nevertheless illustrates the strength of feeling about preserving human life. If, for European Jews, this is taken together with the horror and meaninglessness of the massive numbers of deaths in the Holocaust, it can be seen why the instinct to stay alive is so strong.

Traditionally, orthodox Jews believe in an afterlife, a world to come, though on the whole Jewish tradition has left the precise nature of this afterlife unclear. Orthodox Jews assert in their daily prayers that they believe in such an afterlife, and in the coming of a personal Messiah. Non-orthodox Jews are less clear about an afterlife, and many doubt the idea of a personal Messiah at all. The extent to which Jews genuinely believe these so-called principles of faith is unclear. The experience of the Holocaust has rocked the faith of many Jews in a dramatic fashion, and little research has been done on the precise nature of modern Jewish belief. Suffice it to say that non-orthodox Jews do not tend to believe in a physical afterlife, and many do not believe in an after-life at all.

Yet, despite this, irrespective of belief or lack of it, irrespective of whether a Jew be an agnostic or even an atheist, when it comes to the time to die, many Jews will want to die as Jews. At the very least, it will mean wanting a Jewish funeral of some kind. It may also mean wanting a rabbi or members of a local Jewish community to come in and talk to him or her about a Jewish death and funeral, particularly if the person is someone whose family is mostly not Jewish, who has married someone not Jewish where knowledge of Jewish rituals and beliefs is not great.

But, many Jews will not want to carry out all the rituals listed below. It is as well to ask individuals and their families what they want to do, the key being to make possible everything that they actually do want to do. These things may be observing dietary laws, though they have not always done so in the past, or praying on the Sabbath or on other days of the week. It may be observing festivals, and it may be simply discussing what it means to be a Jew (a common Jewish preoccupation) with other Jews or with people caring for the individual.

On dietary laws, many Jews observe them strictly and other Jews less so or not at all. Orthodox Jews will tend to observe them fairly strictly, and others will vary considerably. However, it is worth knowing the basis of the laws, so that kosher food can be offered, and so that the individual and the family feel that their tradition is being taken seriously, part of the reason for paying attention to all these issues at all. The Jewish dietary laws consist in only eating meat that is kosher (it means fit) which, in a healthcare setting, means buying in kosher meals from the kosher meals service. Kosher meat has been killed according to Jewish law, and it has then been soaked to get rid of the blood. Jews also do not eat any animal that does not have a cloven hoof and chew the cud – hence no pork, and hence the horror of the pig in much Jewish folk-lore, for it was one of the things Jews were forced to eat in order to survive at times of intense persecution. Jews do not eat shellfish either, or any fish with no fins and scales, as well as no bird of prey. But the most important thing to know, partly because it is so complicated, is that those who observe the dietary laws strictly do not mix meat and milk.

As well as dietary laws, many Jews, however ill, perhaps especially because they are, will want to observe the sabbath. That will mean at the least lighting the sabbath candles on the Friday evening as the sabbath begins (it runs from sundown to sundown), praying the sabbath prayers, perhaps having a special meal, if able to cope with it, and not doing anything which might be construed as work, such as using a light switch. (it creates a spark). Again, for many non-Jews, this seems deliberately difficult. Yet, for Jews these matters become fantastically important, and though a sick or dying Jewish person is not required to observe all the laws, since all laws can be broken to save life, bar three, nevertheless many Jews in such a situation will want to carry them out in full detail. Hence, healthcare staff should not be surprised if their Jewish patients are lying in the dark on a Friday evening but do not ask directly to have the light put on. It is still a kindness to turn on lights and turn them off again for an orthodox Jew who is trying to observe his or her religion.

Similarly with the High Holy Days, the most solemn days of the year. New Year is the beginning of the penitential season, when real repentance starts and when a Jew is expected to ask forgiveness from those whom he or she has offended, and ask forgiveness of God for sins against God. And the Day of Atonement, Yom Kippur, is the culmination of all this, and Jews fast on it, and stay in the synagogue all day.

Plainly, someone who is dying cannot do all this. Jewish law does not require that someone ill should do so anyway. But many terminally ill Jews prefer to do it. It is, in their view, their last chance. They want to fast. They know it will be hard. Sometimes staff can help with this, including when a dying person does not want to take his or her drugs. For Yom Kippur is the day when even the least religious, the least attentive, of Jews go to the synagogue, and, for those who cannot because they are dying, this day on which we remember our mortality most particularly has a bitter ring, and many people will want to mark it in some way, whether by reading Psalms or saying prayers from the liturgy or simply by fasting, and staying away from drugs is immaterial.

Last rites and funeral customs

In Judaism, when death is very near, Psalms are read and the dying person is encouraged to say the first line of a prayer called the Shema (Hear, O Israel, the Lord is our God, the Lord is one) as his dying words. There is also an opportunity for private confession, not spoken, and for all assembled to gather together for Psalms. After the death, there is much to be done. Jews want no delay in the funeral, liking if possible to have the burial conducted within 24 hours of the death, or 48 hours at worst. (Jews and Muslims often feel disgusted at the sorts of week-long delays before funerals they see for Christians amongst whom they live. They also argue that it is impossible to begin to grieve properly if one is still waiting for the funeral.) There is considerable resistance to post mortem examinations for that reason (and others), and it is preferred for the body to remain intact without the removal of vital organs, although some less orthodox Jews are committed organ donors. The usual insistence on burial does not always apply, since non-orthodox (Reform and Liberal, commonly grouped together as Progressive) allow cremation, though the preference still tends to be for burial.

When a death occurs, people stay by the body for eight minutes whilst a feather is left over the nose and mouth to check if breathing has completely stopped. The eyes and mouth are then closed by the son or nearest relative, the arms extended down by the sides of the body and the jaw bound up before rigor mortis sets in. Traditionally, the body is then placed on the floor with its feet towards the door, covered with a sheet, with a candle beside it, and not left alone until burial. This cannot fit in with the routine of most hospitals and hospices, but the body may be removed to a side room where it can remain until the sexton comes to collect it. It should be made clear that, unless the family has given express permission, the staff should not attempt to lay out the body.

Jews do not, in general, leave a body alone, and there is a system of watchers (called wachers) staying by the body, reciting Psalms. Many congregations also have a group called the chevra kaddisha (holy assembly) of men and women who wash and prepare the bodies for the funeral, an act considered to be a great honour. After the funeral, the family return home and the chief mourners sit on low stools (called shiva chairs after the shiva, seven days of mourning with evening prayers in the home at which the community come to join in the prayers, pay their respects to the mourners and comfort them). Ritual food is eaten, usually hard-boiled eggs, bagels and lentils or beans, things which are round to symbolise the roundness of life. Prayers are held for seven nights, and people come bearing gifts of food. The mourners do not shave, and they wear slippers or shoes not made of leather, as well as having a tear in their clothes to symbolise the ancient custom of ripping clothes in grief (which itself took the place of ripping the flesh in grief). After the seven nights, there is lesser mourning for 30 days (shloshim) with no festivities and daily trips to the synagogue to say kaddish, the mourners' prayer, and then 11 months of lesser mourning until the consecration of the tombstone and the beginning of picking up the threads of life again, after a full cycle of a year.

Hints for healthcare professionals

In order to help Jewish patients and relatives to have a 'good death', knowing something about their beliefs and practices is only one part of what is required. Obviously one can then offer to provide certain things. But, more important than that, is the willingness to know enough in order to ask – whether it be a relative, or a patient, a friend or someone who is acting as a volunteer sitter for a hospice at home scheme. People need to be asked how much they wish to observe, how much they wish to do, what they actually want done when they die. Nothing will replace asking the questions, provided an opening is given which makes it clear that the person knows that he or she is dying. And asking the questions may bring forth a torrent of answers, some of which may seem to be curiously unrelated to the question asked, and more to do with the individual's relationship with the Jewish community. But those are important worries, concerns and resentments often to be got out of the way. It is only by asking the question that one can find out how orthodox, how traditional, the person was, and establish what would really help at the time of the death, or just before or just after.

When the death occurs, the nurses should ideally not touch the body. If, however, the body has to be touched, it should merely be for the arms to be straightened, the mouth closed, and the body wrapped in a simple white sheet. Everything else will be done by the community itself, and it is much appreciated if the healthcare professionals, where there is no family available, can contact a local synagogue relatively quickly after a death.

Whilst other faiths, different from Christianity, have their rituals which have some similarities with each other, there is a real line to be drawn between Christianity, Islam and Judaism on the one hand and the religions of the Indian sub-continent on the other – the religions that started their lives in India and Tibet. For instance, Buddhism, though now very popular in the west, is essentially an eastern religion, as is Hinduism and Sikhism; and Islam, though it has huge numbers of adherents in the Indian sub-continent, is in fact a middle-eastern religion in origin and different in kind from Hinduism and Buddhism, having more in common with some aspects of Sikhism.

Sikhism

Sikhism is a religion of increasing international importance, and its adherents are usually easily recognised by their wearing of the turban and the other four signs of Sikhism.

History

There is great controversy amongst academic historians of religion who say that Sikhism is either an offshoot of Hinduism or that it is Hinduism heavily influenced by Islam. In fact, neither is wholly true. It is, in a sense, an offshoot of Hinduism in that it grew up amongst people who had previously been Hindus. But, they became strongly disaffected from it, regarding some parts of it as positively dangerous, and other elements as unnecessarily ritualistic.

The Sikh religion is monotheistic and was founded by Guru Nanak (1469–1533). Sikh means disciple or follower, and it is as followers of Guru Nanak and his nine successors that the Sikhs became an independent religious body.

Guru Nanak had been born a Hindu, and was shocked by many of the features of contemporary Hinduism. He particularly deplored the caste system and the power and influence of the priesthood. His aim was to return to the essentials of religion, to the relationship of each individual with his God, to the search for a virtuous life, and to the idea that only by doing good in this life was there a route to salvation. Much of this is highly individual and personal, there being a strong element of personal religion within Sikhism as each individual strives to know God. There is a strong community aspect to Sikhism as well, and the life of the community in the gurdwara (Sikh temple), where all Sikhs gather, is seen as one of group activity, especially eating together. Guru Nanak had nine successors, finishing with Guru Gobind Singh, who consolidated his work. The book of Sikhism is the Guru Granth Sahib, which terminally ill Sikhs often want to hear read aloud. Community action is the mode by which Sikhism operates; there is no priesthood. The gurdwara is a centre of learning and of prayer, of eating together and hospitality. It is also the source of help for any Sikh in distress, and where once travellers and the homeless stayed, and indeed still sometimes can stay.

Specific beliefs and customs

The symbols of Sikhism are the kesh, uncut hair, usually worn in a bun by both men and women and covered with the characteristic turban which all Sikh men wear, and a few elderly pious Sikh women as well. Then there is the kangha, the comb, worn in the hair, which will be kept with them even if for some reason, say radiotherapy or chemotherapy, it cannot be attached to the hair because the hair has fallen out. There is the kara, the steel bangle, which once again all Sikhs wear, and which they will want to have taped to their arm if they have to have surgery, where in other circumstances such a bangle might be removed. There is the kirpan, the symbolic dagger, the symbol which has caused more difficulties in the healthcare setting than I would have believed possible. The kirpan is rarely a large sword ready for military action, though that is its role, since the Sikhs were warrior people. It is now usually a few inches long, blunt and useless. Nevertheless, hospital staff particularly tend to get upset seeing some kind of knife on the bedclothes, so that usually it is a good idea for the family to explain. In fact, in the UK, most Sikhs wear a brooch or some other pin or pendant, and it is not a real dagger at all. Lastly there are the kaccha, the special underpants or shorts. Sikhs never completely remove their underwear. They shower or bath with one leg in the old pair, before putting on the new pair as they remove the old one. It seems highly complicated for many friends and staff, but it is extremely important to most Sikhs, being bound up, almost certainly, with ideas of modesty, of sexuality, and being invented probably to replace the dhoti, a length of cloth wound round the legs, to make for easier movement in times of war, the Sikhs being a war-like group.

Sikhism has no clear belief in an afterlife. It is very much orientated towards a this-life approach, and to this world. It has a disciplined approach to life, and Sikhs are supposed to be involved with family, friends and community rather than following the sometimes ascetic, very often other-worldly, disciplines of Hinduism. Like Hindus, Sikhs tend to believe in a series of reincarnations, which means they often have very little difficulty in accepting forthcoming death. Each soul goes through cycles of rebirth, so that death causes no fear. The ultimate objective is for each soul to reach perfection, to be reunited with God and not to have to re-enter this world. Despite the concentration in much of Sikh thought on this world, this life, the doctrine of the karma remains, so that each person's present life is influenced by his actions in the last life, and the actions of this life set the scene for what will happen in the next life, and so on.

The major difference, which has important psychological and social consequences, is that unlike Hindus, Sikhs believe that the cycle can be altered by exceptionally virtuous actions. They believe in the power of the individual, and in the extension of God's grace. At the time of the death, therefore, they tend not to be particularly frightened, and will welcome readings from the Guru Granth Sahib, organised by the local gurdwara or the family, as well as opportunities for private prayer.

Last rites and funeral customs

When the death happens, a Sikh is cremated as quickly as possible, in India within 24 hours. In Britain, this is harder to achieve, although, like with Muslims and Jews, funerals are often arranged within 48 hours, and after the cremation the ashes are taken to India and eventually scattered over the river Sutlej in Anandpur, in the Punjab, where Sikhism was founded. Although there is little to debate in attitudes to funerals and speed in having the cremation, sometimes Sikhs want to talk about whether they want their ashes scattered in the Punjab, since increasingly they want their ashes in their gardens in England, or wherever. This can be a matter of debate, as can whether the traditional mourning procedures will be gone through. For, after the funeral, there is usually some kind of funeral meal at the gurdwara, and often women do not eat until the cremation has taken place. After 10 days or so, there is a ceremony to mark the end of the first stage of formal mourning, rather like in Judaism, entitled Bhog. The Guru Granth Sahib is read in full either at home or at the gurdwara, and this reading marks the end of the formal mourning period so that life can go back, as far as is possible, to normal. This is sometimes not wanted by Sikhs who are dying, although many Sikhs want the most traditional of marking of their deaths. Those who are not Sikhs but are helping to care for a Sikh patient who is near the end need to realise just how community-based Sikhism is. Whilst Sikhs are usually extremely happy to explain their religion and to include people who are not Sikhs into their ceremonies, it is the community which matters, and community visitors, and community plans for the funeral that will be central to the dying person's concerns.

Hints for healthcare professionals

The most important thing to remember when caring for a Sikh patient is just how important the five signs of Sikhism are. For instance, nursing help which allows a Sikh patient who has had, or is having, extensive chemotherapy and losing his or her hair, to keep the hair attached to the head with a series of hairnets of different meshes and overlapping is very welcome. Similarly, anything which allows the steel bangle to be worn whatever treatment is being given, or procedure carried out in an operating theatre, say by taping it to the wrist, is very much appreciated, as is attaching the dagger, the kirpan, to the body in some way. Indeed, the most important thing someone caring for a Sikh patient can do is show respect to the symbols and make it as easy as possible for them to keep them with them.

The other thing is to realise just how community-based Sikhism is, and how likely it is that many members of the community will be there with a dying person. In hospices, and in some hospitals, sometimes the sheer number and presence of people reading the Guru Granth Sahib can be overwhelming, but healthcare professionals can explain what is going on to other patients, and can even arrange a private room where necessary.

Hinduism

Hinduism is a thoroughly misunderstood religion in Britain. It is perceived as polytheistic, and somehow pagan, unlike the three 'great' religions of Judaism, Christianity and Islam which are monotheistic. This often means that Hindus, when seriously ill and deserving of the full gamut of spiritual care from staff and friends, do not get it. Their religion is not seen as 'real', their faith leads to impossible miracles like statues drinking milk, but is not about the important things of life: sin, atonement, salvation, faith, charity.

This is deeply offensive, and, of course, untrue. It is really important that we should do better by our Hindu patients than we have. Many serious experts on religious history and theory argue that Hinduism is no more polytheistic than Judaism or Islam – indeed, that Christianity's treatment of Jesus and the Holy Spirit with the 'three in one' theory may be more polytheistic – and that the various deities are in fact all ramifications of the one true eternal being, the creator god, who is expressed in a variety of different ways. Thus Brahma, the creator, Vishnu, the preserver, and Shiva, the destroyer and regenerator of life, are, in a sense, all part of one and the same. And all the other gods, Rama and Krishna as incarnations of Vishnu, and so on, are all ramifications of his one being.

History

Hinduism is more than a religion. Some argue that it is a series of '-isms', a collection of different, very early religions somehow taken over and incorporated into one. Others say that it is a way of life, and that that way of life has itself varied from place to place. It is practised fairly widely in Britain. There are active Hindu societies in many of our big cities, and there are Hindu temples and cultural groups.

Hinduism is a very ancient religion; no-one is certain of its exact age. It has thousands of gods and goddesses, but most Hindus would argue that these are all manifestations of one god in many different forms. There is, quite understandably, some resentment amongst Hindus in Britain that their religion is not taken sufficiently seriously by people of other faiths, and it is important to understand something of the Hindu pantheon.

The three supreme gods of Hinduism are Brahma, the creator, Vishnu the preserver, and Shiva the destroyer and regenerator of life. But with these go innumerable other gods; anyone who has ever been to India will have seen the figures, statuettes and pictures of local or particularly helpful gods: Ganesh, the elephant god, frequently on the front of lorries; Kali, Shiva's wife, at the back of shops in the bazaar.

Hindus divide up into different sects, whose beliefs and philosophies are quite different. The majority of Hindus in Britain are Vishnavites, that is to say that they worship principally Vishnu the preserver and his incarnations as Rama and Krishna. As Rama, Vishnu was a good king, combining beauty, bravery and justice. As Krishna, he was a charming young man who brought with him happiness and fun as well as power and justice. Some Vishnavites believe that he will come again in a future incarnation as Kaliki, when he will bring about the end of the world and destroy evil forever. Most Hindu religious literature dates from three or four millennia ago at the earliest: there are the Vedas, the Upanishads, the Brahmanas, and the long epics of the Bhagavad Gita, based on the Nahabharata, and the Ramayana.

Hinduism has its origin in India and is largely practised by people of Indian origin, but it is an international, world religion now, with temples all over the world, and growing interest in its philosophies and its healthcare practices in the western world.

Specific beliefs and customs

The Hindu view of life is one we need to understand if we are to help someone who is a believing and observant Hindu to die well. For Hindus divide life up into: brahmacharya, the time of education; garhasthya, the time of working in the world; vanapastha, the time for loosening worldly ties and worldly attachments; and, finally, pravrajya or yati, awaiting freedom through death. Life is staged. Hindus expect to wait for death. It holds little fear, except insofar as the process of dying might be unpleasant. This is fundamentally different from a Christian who may fear hellfire and damnation, even now, or a Jew who fears the nothingness that death might well bring. But reaching the stage of renunciation and readiness for death is to be done gracefully. Those of us involved in caring for Hindus in such a position should help to achieve that sense of grace, and to maintain it, which is not always easy.

Hindus believe in reincarnation. They will return to earth either in a better or worse form, according to their karma. Karma is much misunderstood in the west. It is not pure unadulterated fatalism. What a person does in this life will affect what happens to them in the next. Similarly, the position and life in this world is seen as, at least in part, a reflection on what the person did in a previous life. To add to that, and significantly for those of us concerned with caring for someone who is a Hindu, health and well-being in this life can often be thought to be the reward for living by the moral laws. Hinduism is not alone in presenting this view. The Hebrew Bible is full of threats by God to give a short life to sinners and promises to give a long life to those who follow God's law. But such thinking is very difficult. How can one explain the death of a small child who cannot yet have done very much at all? What does it mean for some people to be smitten, by chance, with some rare and fatal disease? Or simply to live as poor people in the path of an oncoming flood?

There is, too, alongside all this a view of Hindu medicine, Ayurvedic medicine, which contains a well-defined discipline of good healthcare different from our own western attitude to health. Ayurvedic medicine can be combined with western medicine, but not necessarily very easily. Yet, the routine recommended to its followers is a regular diet, sleep, defecation, cleanliness of body and clothing, and moderation in physical exercise and sexual indulgence. It is a little bit along the lines of 'moderation in all things', but linked to a disciplined view of the world, and of how one should live one's daily life. Much of it should therefore fit all too well with the western view that moderation in, say, alcohol consumption, is the way to live a healthy life.

Like many groups who originate in the Indian sub-continent or the Middle East, Hindus have strict modesty requirements. No-one caring for them can do anything but respect the immense modesty of many Hindu women, particularly. But this can lead to immense complications when finding out about the genitourinary and bowel areas. Constipation is of course a common problem when people are dying, often a side-effect of pain-relieving drugs being used. Hinduism rules that a doctor cannot attend a woman if her husband is not present. Equally, a woman will not talk about that area of her body if her husband is present. This can cause considerable confusion and distress, and is something that anyone involved in caring for a Hindu person who is dying should watch out for.

There are also rules about ritual purification, and most Hindus will try to bathe every day in running water, so that anyone caring for a Hindu who is dying should try to ensure that that bathing is made possible, even at home when normally a district nurse might come to help with a bath once a week rather than daily. For the thinking behind such bathing is that it renders one spiritually clean as well as physically.

There are also bans on beef for all Hindus, on any kind of meat for many Hindus, especially the women, and, in some cases, on eating food which has been prepared by a Hindu of a different caste from the person concerned, even though the caste system is technically illegal in India these days. There are nevertheless many legacies of it, of which this is merely one which gets noticed more than the others.

Last rites and funeral customs

Most Hindus will spend much of their last days and weeks in prayer and contemplation. Hinduism is a genuinely spiritual approach to God, and the desire for quiet contemplation is very strong. There is also likely to be some Ganges water in a pot beside the bed. This is because the river Ganges, particularly at Varanasi (Benares) is where the burning ghats with the corpses of dead Hindus float, and the Ganges water is a signal both of mortality and of the intention to be disposed of properly. Yet, in fact, most Hindus dying in Britain will be cremated here, with perhaps some Ganges water to hand. Ashes may well be scattered on the Ganges later on, since it is considered the proper place to end up.

In all this, the Hindu priests, the pandits, or Brahmins, can be very helpful. They help dying people with their acts of prayer, called puja. They discuss the philosophical acceptance of death. They talk about reincarnation. Death is accepted without the anger so characteristic of western families.

After the death, the person is cremated, and there is a ceremony called Sreda for the mourners, where food offerings are brought to the Brahmins who then perform some particular rituals for the dead. The mourners will be apart for a while after a death, yet signals of comfort are often physical. Hands are held, hugs are exchanged, in order to give physical comfort to the survivors.

Hints for healthcare professionals

Often we give the wrong kind of care to Hindus whom we are trying to care for. We fail to recognise the fatalism of their outlook, and wait for anger where it does not come. At the same time, we fail to understand that the desire for pain relief is just as strong whether people make a big fuss or are eternally patient, though suffering. It would be good to see Hindus better cared for throughout our healthcare system, with their particular attitudes recognised, pain relief provided, but consciousness in no way impaired, for their desire is often to pray and be spiritually aware.

It is important to recognise that the small figurines of gods can be very helpful placed by the bed of someone who is dying, or a flask of water from the Ganges – a reminder of the final resting home of the body or, more likely in the UK, the ashes, of the person who is dying. Equally, any help with getting a pandit, the Hindu priest, to come is often very welcome. In most large cities, there is a Hindu society and its members are always keen to come and give support to a fellow Hindu in need.

Buddhism

Buddhism is growing rapidly in the west, and has a huge number of adherents throughout the world. However, their practices are very varied. Although they all centre themselves on the discipline of Siddhartha Gautama, and his revelation of four truths, after which he was called Buddha, their similarities are limited to the absence of a godhead and a search for a disciplined life.

Buddhism is still growing rapidly in Britain, a religion, or perhaps series of religious approaches to life, which have particularly found a place in the belief systems of people in their mid-to-late forties and early fifties. Some of this is a result of the swinging sixties and the experimentation with contemplation and transcendent meditation of the seventies. But much of that was synthetic, and the adherents of that time left Buddhism behind, if they had ever really discovered it. Yet Buddhism is the major religion in Burma, Bhutan, Nepal, Sikkim, Sri Lanka, Thailand and Tibet. It is also found increasingly in India, parts of Africa and Japan, and in the west.

History

Buddhism was founded on the Indian sub-continent about 2500 years ago by Siddartha Gautama (an Indian prince), probably in what is now Nepal. He was born in about 560 BC and became deeply troubled by the miseries of life amongst the ordinary people around him in India. He decided to try to help his people find happiness and contentment by searching for truth. The answer (or perhaps more accurately the beginning of the answer) was the four noble truths which Gautama discovered as he sat on a river bank under a sacred fig tree. From that point on he was called Buddha, which means the enlightened or awakened one.

Buddhism is a unique religion in that it acknowledges no God as creator. It does, however, acknowledge many gods, though these are all seen as lesser beings than the Buddha himself. Some scholars would argue that it is more a way of living than a religion because of its lack of belief in a godhead. Yet it is clearly a religious discipline, with a compelling philosophy. Its teaching is based on non-violence and brotherhood, with a duty incumbent on its adherents to seek spiritual growth. Buddhists believe in a doctrine of rebirth – often thought, mistakenly, by westerners to be the same as reincarnation. In the Buddhist rebirth, everything changes when an individual who has lived many lives before carries on into a future life after death. But, whatever someone does in this particular present life influences the next stage in the rebirth process. If the individual pays attention to the teachings of Buddhism and tries to live by them, then in each life he learns from past experiences and gradually progresses towards perfection, nirvana. The achievement of nirvana implies the reaching of the infinite state of perfection where there is no selfishness, and no awareness of one's own separate identity. At the same time, there should be no repression of one's true need for personal spiritual growth. Some people stayed with Buddhism and worked at it seriously. They, along with other people who came to it slightly later, are the core of modern Buddhist movements in Britain, some of which have been instrumental in promoting inter-faith discussion, and global co-operation.

Buddhists in Britain are members of all the different schools of Buddhism which exist. There is Theravada Buddhism, usually a bit stricter than other forms, and Mahayyana Buddhism, the so-called 'Greater Way'. There is also Zen Buddhism, an offshoot of Mahayyana Buddhism originally, which was brought by a Buddhist teacher from India, Bodhidharma, to China in around 520 AD. Zen Buddhism comes from the Japanese translation of the Chinese word chan, which was from the Sanskrit dhyana, which means meditation. Zen Buddhism has a rich diet of meditation, as well as a strong influence on Japanese martial arts, and samurai warrior skills. Some people find it strange that Buddhism of any kind, with its essentially peaceful approach to life, should be so influential in martial arts. But Zen Buddhism has also influenced the Japanese tea ceremony, a formal and peaceful activity, as well as Japanese flower arranging, and formal gardening. It is, too, a very intellectual approach to Buddhism, requiring a considerable intellectual discipline which has found much in the way of adherence in academic communities in the western world.

Specific beliefs and customs

There is a doctrine of rebirth in Buddhism, somewhat different from that in Hinduism and Sikhism, for everything changes as the individual progresses from one life to the next. It is possible to observe the teachings of the Buddha and to live such a good life that one gradually approaches nirvana, perfection, where selfishness is gone and separate identity is no more. There is a rigorous discipline which recognises that human existence and suffering are inextricably linked, and which demands of its adherents a gradual heightening of the awareness of the spirit, where physical realities matter less and less, leading to a state of perfect freedom and peace.

Buddhism is unusual amongst the world's religions in that it does not acknowledge a personal god as a creator at all. The Buddhist is expected to make his or her way to a form of 'nirvana', perfection, perfect peace and freedom without suffering, through his or her own actions. There is an eight-fold path which a Buddhist is expected to take, and meditation, and the development of self-discipline, is the way to go along this path. Various disciplines are used to go along the eightfold path, and to try to reach nirvana, and some of these will be practised by Buddhists who are terminally ill.

The Buddhist view of life and death, with the body only a temporary vessel but often with strict views about how it should be used, is different from a western one. Indeed, often Buddhist attitudes are more difficult for westerners to understand and accept than those found in Hinduism or Sikhism. There is something in most Buddhist world views about death not mattering in its physical ramifications. The next world is to be prepared for; it can be looked forward to with a kind of equanimity rare in, say, western Christianity. Buddhist sisters and brothers seem to bring comfort as they help a Buddhist to pray and meditate, and the preparation for death includes the usual acceptance of cremation, conducted sometimes by a member of the family, or a Buddhist bhikku (monk) or sister. Calmness is the hallmark of the dying Buddhist – or, at least, it should be. It seems very different from the attitude shown by adherents of other faiths or members of other communities.

However, there are Buddhists who experience extreme pain, or who find meditation impossible in the circumstances. Often, they feel they are being bad Buddhists. They are not behaving properly, not attempting the discipline that is the central core of Buddhism.

Hints for healthcare professionals

For those of us caring for Buddhists who feel like this, there are great difficulties. We can often sympathise with their reactions, for they are much more like the reactions of people of other faiths to their impending death. There is anger instead of calm, there is fear of pain, there is grief, there is denial. But we tread carefully, because the Buddhist who goes through all this feels that he or she should not be doing so. They feel somehow inadequate, failures. We should support them as best we can, and assure them that other people go through the same stages of anger and grief, but we should also let them call in a bhikku or sister, to discuss the issues with them. For Buddhism can be very hard, and those who have become Buddhists in adult life, having started from a Christian background, often find older attitudes, or cultural attitudes of western ways, coming to the top of their consciousness. We have to tread very carefully here, because if a Buddhist wants to die well, he or she wants no part of the common patterns of grief that western psychologists have recognised and described.

So helping Buddhists come to the good death, to die well, is far from easy. It sets us a real challenge. Buddhists have a very different world view, one that many of us cannot quite understand. And they find what many westerners regard as acceptable and normal to be a weakness of spirit. Yet we encourage others to show their emotions along this scale of gradually changing stages of grief. We need to tread carefully, and be enormously sensitive, as well as asking questions of the individual about what he or she would really like to help them come to terms with the situation, be it time for meditation, a visit from a bhikku, or just the chance to talk to us about what they feel.

For instance, a Buddhist who is dying will require as much time and space for meditation as is practically possible. Many Buddhists will refuse all forms of pain-controlling drugs because they wish to reach the stage of ultimate awareness, which is not possible if they are in any way drugged or in any way without every possible physical and mental sensation. Buddhism stresses the importance of the relief of pain and suffering in general, which makes the reaction by many Buddhists to pain-relieving drugs quite difficult to deal with. Yet, if we want to help the Buddhist to achieve his or her version of 'the good death', we must recognise that their attitudes to pain relief and to the possibility of having a clouded mind are very different from some other people's. All that can be done is to assure the person, if it is true, that their mind will be in no way clouded by the drugs. That, in itself, requires very careful titration of drug doses, and means that staff in a professional situation caring for a Buddhist who is dying will have to be very certain of their own capabilities.

Chinese customs

There are many many groups, cultural and religious communities, in Britain. I have only scratched the surface. To these can be added Chinese customs, though many Chinese people will be Christian and others Buddhist, and still others Confucian. As with all other groups, it is essential not to generalise about the Chinese. This is particularly important since so many different religions can be found in China, as well as a strong Communist tradition of anti-religious feeling, which has not succeeded in removing many of the traditions associated with earlier religious faiths. Suffice it to say that, in most of south China, it is hard to say where Taoism ends and Buddhism begins in relation to death and other life-cycle events, and it is also clearly common for Chinese Christians to practice some of the same rituals as their Buddhist and Taoist neighbours.

History

The separation of religion by class is worth noting. The scholars and gentry tended to be Confucian, which is more a philosophy than a religion, with its emphasis on solving the practical difficulties of everyday life in an ethical way. Heaven is a universal moral law, a cosmic order. There is no sense of sin, human nature is essentially good, and evil comes about as a result of humans doing bad things, often under the influence of their leaders.

Meanwhile, the ordinary people developed a folk religion, which then became supplemented by, and indeed combined with, Taoism and Buddhism. Folk religion is alive with spirit gods, kitchen gods and earth gods. The gods have magical powers and are much feared, as well as being frequently bought off or placated. Festivals such as Chinese New Year are closely tied in with the folk religion. But it is practised by people who are Taoist or Confucian, Buddhist and Christian as well, even though it is all tied up with astrology, with palm-reading, with dream interpretation and other magical practices.

Taoism has its roots in the writings of Lao-Tzu, and has the central concept of the development of inner peace and certainty being possible if people centre their way of life on the way of the universe or the dao. Through contemplation of nature, one's deepest and most human expectations can surface from the artificial expectations of society. Taoist priests teach breath control, exercises similar to Hatha yoga, and also use a variety of potions and elixirs to delay or prevent death. The prevalence of Taoism has much diminished, but traditional Chinese medicine still relies heavily on the Taoist traditions.

But central to all Chinese religions is a mixture of folk religion and the family. If Chinese society is to be a moral society, then the place to start is in the family. Ancestors were worshipped, and are still respected now. It is believed that the spirits of ancestors are capable of punishing moral offenders, and also rewarding good behaviour. Belief in life after death, a key part of all Chinese religions, is strengthened by the building of altars to ancestors and placing spirit tablets on them, which one often sees in the room of a dying person of a Chinese family.

Specific beliefs and customs

This universal belief in ancestors is particularly complicated since more fanatical Chinese Christians will cheerfully refer to Taoism and Buddhism as 'Devil worship', a strange ascription to be given to the followers of Buddha and Confucius. Nevertheless, it is important to realise that, despite religious variation, and even religious enmity, many of the rituals will remain the same.

Amongst these is the fatalism surrounding an impending death and the desire to be prepared for it. So as soon as it becomes clear that the person is unlikely to recover, about which no secrets are kept, a coffin has to be procured. Often, coffins are purchased much earlier in life, by children wanting to show their parents that everything proper will be done when the time comes. So it is not uncommon for the dying person to be in the room with his or her own coffin, and for several prayers and blessings to be said which make it clear that the most important thing in life, now ending fast, is to be buried properly with all the necessary pomp and circumstance.

During the process of dying, there are few rituals which are universal. But the concern for propriety after the death is paramount. Although a dying Chinese person may want to see the Buddhist priest or sister, or may want, if Christian, to see the priest, it is often to discuss the funeral arrangements, and to make it clear that the family is to gather around. Once the death has taken place, the body is washed an uneven number of times by family, in special water thought to be protected by a guardian spirit. The ceremony is known as 'buying the water' and, like other religions, the feeling that the body can be, in some way, possessed is very strong, so that incense is burnt at the same time and firecrackers exploded, to keep the evil spirits away. The body is then covered in wadding before it is dressed, another way of keeping the spirits out. The clothing is usually cotton, unless the family is very wealthy, in which case silk is used, and the garments have no buttons or zips, but are tied with fabric ties, so that the clothing looks rather like the clothing of a Buddhist priest. Sometimes, the dying person asks to see the garment before he dies, in order to check that it is in keeping with the solemnity and status required of his death. Men have a similar headdress to the Buddhist priests, whilst women wear the 'Lotus flower hat', a seven-cornered hat with their hair piled high on the head, dressed with gold, or jade. The men often have a jade snuff bottle put in the tomb with them, and the use of jade near the body dates from a very early period.

After being dressed, the body is given socks and shoes, which the dying person also often wishes to see, and is then bound at the feet with a piece of rope, to stop it leaping about if it is attacked by evil spirits. It is then laid out on the bed for friends and family to pay their last respects. A drummer is outside the door, on the left hand side for a man, on the right for a women, to play warning beats as guests approach so that the family can be found in suitable attitudes of mourning, in a formal tableau style.

The coffin is placed on two stools, head pointing to the door, and a table is arranged as an altar, with five vessels on it. There are blue and white paper flowers in the vases, and two candlesticks are lit at night. Alongside these is a pagoda-shaped lamp stand with a bowl of sesame oil, containing a burning wick of twisted cotton. The spirit tablet, which has the name of the deceased person on it, and into which one of his souls has entered, is in the centre of the altar next to the coffin.

There is fairly standard food for the family, but when guests come there is a banquet, and the food is often, at least partly, brought in by the guests themselves, to create a good spread. Once again, the dying person often wishes to be assured that this will take place, even in a community which has few Chinese people in it. For the guests bring gifts which are for the deceased. The gifts include money in a yellow paper envelope, with a strip of blue to indicate mourning. There are also banners which bear the words: 'May the soul return to the Western Heaven', which are carried in the funeral procession and burned after the service of committal. Then, there are gold and silver, paper money, and paper carts and horses, all for burning in the final cortège.

Before the burial, specialists have to be consulted. The religious authorities will gauge the family's wealth and decide just how many masses need to be sung in order to gain entrance to the Western Heaven. The virtues of the dead person are sung aloud, unless he or she was notoriously an evil-doer, in which case the priests have to make intercessions, a form of plea in mitigation, imploring the bad spirits to release the soul of their client. One of the 'adepts' (experts) will determine the best site for the burial, and the diviner is called in to get the spirits of those already buried in the graveyard to agree on the siting. After the masses for the dead person, the family prepares paper offerings representing the things the person was involved in in life, so servants, cars, carts, horses, rickshaws, and so on are all prepared for the deceased's use in the nether world society. On the eve of the funeral these are taken out and burned. Once again, an attendant is there beating at the bonfire with a long pole, to keep any lurking evil spirits away. Boiled rice and water are often scattered to keep the attentions of the Hungry Ghosts away.

On the morning of the funeral, the body is taken out head first, and the youngest son breaks a drinking saucer at its head to give the deceased a drinking vessel in the nether world. Then, there is a proper funeral procession, grouped in multiples of eight; there are banners with eulogies of the deceased and lanterns, flowers and other objects. At intervals along the route, paper money is thrown in the air to distract malignant wandering spirits.

Once they arrive at the cemetery, the coffin is lowered into the grave, the diviner asks the relatives to be certain the place is suitable, and the mourners weep and wail around the grave, and scatter a handful of earth on to the coffin. As the weeping dies down, a bonfire is made of the paper articles at the graveside, and the ceremony comes to an end.

But mourning continues, which a dying Chinese person often wants to ensure will happen. There are ceremonies afterwards for at least 24 hours, and, then, at various auspicious days in the ensuing year. Guests are always welcome at any of these ceremonies, so that those who are friends of a different background are keenly encouraged to join the mourning. It is thought that the presence of someone who is not Chinese, and not a member of the family, gives 'face' (importance) to the deceased, and brings honour to the bereaved family. But it is always as well to check first, though occasionally Chinese patients in terminal care surroundings have made it clear that they would welcome the presence of the staff who have cared for them, even if they are not Chinese, at the funeral or at the feast at the house.

The ceremonies make it clear that death and dying are taken as the culmination of the religious life for many Chinese people, for whom a proper death and funeral is of paramount importance. The concern, therefore, with the funeral arrangements, and with the nature of the coffin, is not to be wondered at.

Hints for healthcare professionals

For caring staff, it is important to realise that this is not morbid obsession but a key part of religious faith. A person who does not have a proper funeral has not lived properly. Similarly, if a person cannot trust his family to provide him with all the ceremonies of honour which a dead Chinese person expects, how can he take their grief at his final sickness seriously? These are concerns which are often voiced at the bedside of a terminally ill Chinese man (more often than with a woman). He wants to know that everything has been organised, and he wants to check that the family knows, and remembers, what to do. There will be a great deal of variation in the ritual which is undertaken, but, in almost all cases, the washing, and the insistence on burial (though exhumation takes place after six years in Hong Kong, and bones are kept in funerary jars), and the requirement of feasting and formal mourning will remain the same. For caring staff, the most helpful thing, as ever, is to encourage the dying person to talk about his or her concerns about what will happen to his body and soul, and to understand that the journey to the Western Heaven is one that is not undertaken easily. Similarly, it is important to realise that these concerns may be mixed in with other religious beliefs, notably those of Buddhism and Christianity, which are described elsewhere in this book. It is the mixture of religious and social customs here that is so difficult for caring staff, brought up in the attitudes of western Christianity which regards itself as one single faith, to take on board.

There are many other groupings which could be described, whose beliefs and customs colour the way they approach their death, as ours do. It is part of the human condition that we are coloured by our upbringing and culture to face death in different ways. Groups that could have been included, but are not, are some south Indian customs, variations of Islam from different parts of the world, and so on, let alone very tiny groups of people from other religions, such as Jains from southern India, Jehovah's Witnesses, really a part of Christianity, and other off-shoots of traditional religions and ancient African and Chinese faith patterns. No chapter on these issues, helping people of different faiths and belief systems and cultural patterns to have a good death according to their lights, can be complete. All it can do is point to some areas of interest, some areas which we need to watch out for, such as modesty and food restrictions, and help to give us just enough basic information to ask questions that will be neither offensive nor disturbing, but enable people who are dying and their families feel that they are being cared for, spiritually as much as physically, and that we wish the dying person to die well according to his or her views, not ours.

But all faiths have a way of bringing the bereaved into the community, including them in action and celebration at some stage, so that, even in the moments of greatest darkness, comfort can be given by the sense of love from a community, as well as from individuals in a family or amongst close friends. For most religious groupings other than Christians in Britain, it is that sense of communal support, in the shape of ritualised grieving, that does bring comfort to the bereaved, and gives people a sense of belonging when a sense of isolation and of loneliness are the most common of emotions.

References

1 Neuberger J (2004) *Caring for Dying People of Different Faiths* (3e). Radcliffe Medical Press, Oxford.
2 Social and Community Planning Research (1992) *British Social Attitudes Survey.* Social and Community Planning Research, Dartmouth.
3 Runnymede Trust Commission on British Muslims and Islamophobia (1997) *Islamophobia: a challenge for us all.* Report of the Runnymede Trust Commission on British Muslims and Islamophobia, London.
4 Suggested by Saba Risaluddin. J Neuberger and J White (eds) (1991) *A Necessary End.* Macmillan, London.

6

How can we make dying better for people?

Is euthanasia an answer?

There are many who say that we could make dying better, easier, for people who are terminally ill by allowing them to slip away painlessly by euthanasia. In other words, once the condition is diagnosed as terminal, the best thing to do would be to get as organised as one can, and then ask a doctor to give one an injection to finish off the business of dying. That view has growing support in parts of the western world. In 1994, British television showed a film about euthanasia Dutch style, where euthanasia in limited circumstances has been decriminalised, and the level of support for such a move, despite the lack of legal backing, was considerable. Increasingly, as state support for the frail elderly decreases, and older people, and their children, see assets diminish at an alarming rate which they had wanted to pass on from genera-tion to generation, the desire to put an end to this grows. When the Labour Government came to power in the UK in 1997, it set up its promised Royal Commission on Long-term Care. But the results of that commission, with a fierce minority report from two dissenters, were that more nursing care became funded in a somewhat haphazard way, but that the cost of long-term care in nursing homes was still the responsibility of individuals or of the local authority if there were insufficient means. Since local authorities were them-selves strapped for cash, this meant very low payments per week for older people in nursing homes, a diminution in standards, and, most worryingly, in large parts of the south east and south west of the UK, a rapid realisation by nursing home owners that more money could be made by selling the property than by continuing to run it as a nursing home. So care of the elderly became a greater and greater political issue in the early years of the new millennium.

It is largely for reasons of property and the fear of gradually becoming destitute whilst paying nursing home fees to be looked after as one nears death, that it has become impossible to discuss the euthanasia issue properly in Britain. The cost of the care of older people has to be borne by them themselves to a very large extent. Yet many of those people had thought that the NHS would indeed look after them from cradle to grave. So, surrounding the issue of the cost of care of the elderly, there is a lot of anger. One way that anger is expressed is by an increasing pressure to allow euthanasia, in order not to waste what one has left on nursing home fees rather than pass it on to one's children.

Yet, of course, that is not an acceptable argument. Difficult though it is to detach the two issues from each other at present in the public mind, it is nevertheless essential to do so. The cost of caring for the frail elderly should not be an argument for legalising, or at least decriminalising, euthanasia. If one goes down that path, then any person who is not economically active, not 'useful' to society, should not be allowed to live. The Nazi extermination of the mentally ill and those with learning difficulties should be a lesson to us all. It is not acceptable to decide to put an end to people because, in some way, they cost the society more than they actually earn for it. That is no way to value human beings.

Assuming, therefore, that no element of the cost of care creeps into the debate, where does the argument for euthanasia lie? For there is undoubtedly a valid argument, although there may be too much on the other side. It lies in the issue of intractable pain, in having a few people whose pain in terminal (and indeed non-terminal) illness is so great that none of the usual ways of dealing with pain touch it at all. There are those involved in palliative care who say that those conditions are very rare, and that they can deal with at least 95% of pain. That may indeed be true. But to be one of the other 5%, the one in 20 whose pain does not respond to the usual treatments, would be very difficult. If one then felt that one's life was one's own, and not in some sense God's gift (which God alone can remove, rather than modern science with a quick, 'end-it-all', injection), there is a legitimate argument for euthanasia. Getting a doctor to put an end to one's misery when one is clearly going to die anyway, and the process is very painful, indeed intolerable, has to be legitimate, morally speaking, for the person who wants to die, if, and only if, they believe their life is their own.

It can equally be an acceptable view for the bystanders. As Sally Vincent put it in *The Guardian* (19 February 1994): 'Dying is our most catastrophic expectation. Not death itself, we hasten to add, but dying. People who have witnessed an agonized and protracted death tend not to develop their experience into a conversation piece. Like a generation of first-world war soldiers, they maintain their trauma in a kind of shamed and unbelieving silence'. They hold the opposite view if they have witnessed a calm and peaceful death, a passing. They wish that it could be like that for everyone, and indeed they talk of watching that as some kind of privilege. In which case, if they so prefer the calm and peaceful passing to the violent and agonised end, it is not surprising if they regard it as something which should be in human control, for them to believe either suicide on the part of the sufferer, or euthanasia, should be allowable, even acceptable.

If one takes that view, then suicide is understandable. One can sympathise with, indeed almost encourage, the person with intractable body pain who decides to make an end of him- or herself. But that is qualitatively different from euthanasia. And that is where the difficulty lies. For even if one does not believe that one's life is one's own to make an end of, as many religious people feel, nevertheless there is a moral objection to asking someone else to do it for you. And it is there that the real objections lie to euthanasia as prac- tised in Holland. For that is not a case of allowing (looking the other way even) someone's suicide. It is not a question of a living will where the carers follow the individual's instructions and cease treatment. Euthanasia demands the active participation of doctors and nurses in the killing of their patients. And, despite the degree of sympathy they may feel for the patients whose lives have become unbearable, the role of healthcare professionals should not be one of actively seeking a person's death. Indeed, the role of the healthcare professional should be to care for the needs of the person whilst alive, and to seek his or her welfare.

Although there are those who would argue that seeking the welfare of someone might mean killing them out of compassion, at their own request, in fact it would be difficult to justify, despite the urge often to give way to the request to put them out of their misery. For the healthcare professionals should be caring or curing. Where cure is impossible, they should be carers. And the nature of that care should be to cherish the life that is there, and not to remove it. Indeed, one of the important values which healthcare profes- sionals have to hold is great respect for human life. It is difficult to retain that respect if one is also prepared to kill one's patients. Yet patients often ask to be killed.

In his book *How we die*, Sherwin Nuland (1994) quotes the example of the Harvard professor of physics, Percy Bridgman, who continued to work until he could no longer do so, aged 79. He was in the last stages of cancer. At his summer home in New Hampshire, he finished the index to the seven volume collection of his scientific works which he had just completed and then went out and shot himself. But he left a suicide note in which he said: 'It is not decent for Society to make a man do this to himself. Probably, this is the last day I will be able to do it myself.' This was not a man who had gone mad. This was not the suicide of the temporarily insane. Percy Bridgman was in his right mind, almost certainly, and he felt he could not bear to go on living, waiting for his imminent and probably unpleasant, undignified, death. He believed that, when the end was inevitable, when he was going to die anyway, even if pain could be relieved, he had a right as a patient to ask his doctor to make an end of him. This is not asking for a doctor to do anything other than anticipating what will happen anyway. He was going to die. It is about making the process faster, painless or nearly so, putting a person out of the misery of a slow and perhaps painful death, allowing them to die with dignity.

Similarly, Hans Kung, probably the greatest theologian of this generation, and Walter Jens in their book *A Dignified Dying: a plea for personal responsibility* make a plea for dignity. They call for human control over human death, with an argument clearly predicated on a belief in human dignity. The underlying theme is that how we die is not necessarily 'natural', or, if 'natural', not necessarily God's will, so it is legitimate to ask for dignity in death. This volume preaches the ultimate desirability of dying peacefully, calmly, in control. Its authors' central Christian belief suggests that a life to come will follow anyway; one can afford to be relaxed about legal protection of every last minute of this life.

Dignity. The word is always used. Dying with dignity. What we all want is to be allowed to die with dignity; hence the other kind of pressure for euthanasia. Because dying well means, for so many of us, dying with dignity, dying decently, tidily, not disintegrating as persons, not being a mess. We do not want to become incontinent if we can avoid it. We do not want to become painfully thin and covered in bedsores. We do not want to have to take so much morphine we will effectively be asleep much of the time, and know little of what is going on around us. We want dignity in our deaths, and the chance to ask our doctors to help us achieve it.

It does not seem to occur to people that there might be something about life that does not allow us that dignity, that to achieve dignity as we die may mean asking doctors to do something more than undignified – in fact, immoral. The debate has raged in many ways in many countries, but the note always in the music is the desire to die with dignity, and Percy Bridgman's feeling that society should not ask people to kill themselves, when doctors could do it so much more easily, and painlessly, and in a dignified way so that one would not have to leave a mess of a shot corpse for someone else to clear up.

But in the end, the debate cannot be about controlling doctors or nurses, or anyone else for that matter. It has to be about whether it is right for healthcare professionals to take life in any circumstance. If it is, then we have to decide when and how, just as we have, vexed though it is, with abortion. And if it is not, then we have to think again about suicide, and how we might make it easier for those who are terminally ill and do not wish to go on, right to the messy end, to commit suicide more easily, more painlessly, with our help but without us carrying out the killing. And it might be worth reflecting that the Dutch Reformed Church in Holland has distinguished between ordinary suicide, out of despair or such like at some other point in one's life, and the kind of suicide, or indeed the Dutch version of euthanasia which they call more or less self-deathing, zelfdoding. The usual word is zelfmoord, self-murder.

Or we could take the view that all this is wrong, and that human beings, patients, must meet their end in whatever way they will, as much as possible without pain, but without having anyone to help them commit suicide, and not having anyone kill them. In the end, they must die at the appropriate time, and we are only obliged to care for them, not kill them.

That means, for many of them, an absence of dignity. Certainly, watching the life of many people in accident and emergency departments, in wards around the country, one does not get the impression of everyone dying with dignity. There is little dignified about an intubated, mechanical death. There is little dignified about a death at the end stages of cancer, painfully thin, often sick as a dog from now pointless chemotherapy. Where diseases cannot be arrested, it seems to me we make it hard if we strive too much to keep people alive, but that is different from active euthanasia.

Yet one can also feel great sympathy for those healthcare professionals who are asked time and again by their patients to put an end to their misery. In 1995, a doctor in Winchester, Nigel Cox, was asked repeatedly by one of his patients who was dying anyway, and in great pain, to put her out of her misery. Over the years, he and his patient had become friends. She trusted him. Her family knew what she was asking. He gave her an injection, and wrote it up in the notes. As it happened, what he gave was so clearly extraordinary that it was obvious something strange was going on. He was reported by the nursing staff. But attitudes have changed. He was not struck off. He was not convicted of murder. He was required to do specific training in pain relief, on the basis that he should have been able to control her pain better. But the general sweep of public sympathy was with him. He had killed his patient with the best of motives, because she had asked him to, because he knew her well and knew when she was serious, and when he knew she was dying anyway. Where, the public felt, was the harm in that?

Passive euthanasia

Indeed, there are those who argue that other cases, such as that of the young man Tony Bland injured in the Hillsborough football stadium disaster, who ended up in a persistent vegetative state (PVS) and for whom a decision had to be made about whether to continue to feed him, are much more cruel. If it was felt that he would never be conscious again, and that he knew nothing of what was going on, if it was felt that there was no point continuing his life, why then should he be starved to death, and deprived of liquids, rather than simply given an injection to end his life? Is it really legitimate to describe cessation of feeding as withdrawal of treatment, and giving an injection to kill him, in that situation, as murder? The judges plainly thought so, and the Tony Bland case cannot be used as a precedent. Each case of that ilk will have to go to court for an application to cease feeding. Yet the decision to stop feeding does pose major moral issues, particularly about the nature of the distinction between cessation of feeding and actually ending a person's life quickly and humanely. It could be argued (and of course was) that feeding a person is part of one's natural duty towards them anyway. To argue that somehow cessation of feeding is not an abrogation of one's duty to them, but that killing them when they have no real life anyway is morally wrong, is difficult to justify. Yet that is the situation we are in, at present, in Britain when debating these issues.

Sally Vincent, in her *Guardian* piece on the subject, just before the House of Lords were debating euthanasia in 1994, cited the case of a friend whose father had a massive stroke and was admitted to hospital. He was 92, and the consultant told his daughter that her father's brain damage was irreversible, and gave her his best advice, which was for the hospital to stop feeding and medicating her father. If that were allowed, he would be physically as well as mentally dead in 19 days. The daughter went back to her father and sat beside him and held his hand. She felt the resources being used to care for her father could be used on someone younger, more deserving, more likely to recover. She knew he had had a long and good life. She knew she would not want to lie there lingering on, and nor would he. She pressed his hand and tried to imagine a response from him. And then he sneezed. She knew his sneeze. It was in her father's voice. She knew it was an involuntary spasm, but it was in her father's tone of voice. So she decided that she did not want her father to starve to death, even if he would not know anything about it, because she did not want to see him waste away, nor drown in his own lung fluid.

She felt the disapproval, the general air of impatience. But her father died seven days later, without being starved, of natural causes. She felt she had done the right thing, though she knew decisions like this, about euthanasia in a passive manner, are being made all the time in our hospitals. Her sense that her father's voice was still there in his sneeze, and that, in any case, he had paid his dues, so what was the hurry, he was going to die anyway, prevented her from saying yes. But how often is the decision made without reference to a daughter who hears the sneeze, a son who still feels the pressure of a bony hand, or whatever?

Advance directives

A way through?

It is, at least in part, because of all this that many are arguing for a legally enforceable 'living will' or advance directive. The UK government is proposing legislating for advance directives during the course of 2004. Yet, in one sense, such advance directives already exist. We sign them when we give consent to surgery, allowing the surgeon to do what he or she sees fit, given what they find. Ever since the beginning of the AIDS epidemic there have also been many young men who have made advance directives about how they wish to be treated when the time comes at the very end of their lives, and the Terrence Higgins Trust has piloted a form of advance directive which others have used, partly as a result of disquiet about intensive, hi-tech care at the end of life.

In Britain, in Europe generally, the debate is not mostly about hi-tech care. But people still want to make advance directives. They still want to be able to say that, if they get Alzheimer's disease, they do not want intense efforts made to keep them alive. They still want to say that they do not wish to go into intensive care if they are in a state where they are unlikely to recover full intellectual capabilities. They do not want to be kept alive as 'vegetables', as the expression goes. They want to be allowed to die 'with dignity', and that means less intervention, not more, and good pain relief and emotional support. But the gradual move towards advance directives, with the House of Lords Committee on medical ethics looking at both this and euthanasia, with a private members' bill introduced into the House of Lords by Lord Joffe in 2003, means that, increasingly, individuals will be able to make some of those important decisions in advance. Indeed, we should encourage people to do so. There is the argument that suggests one cannot tell what one will feel like if one has got Alzheimer's, and what seemed intolerable earlier would seem quite pleasant 30 years on. There is also evidence that suggests that people change a great deal in what they regard as an acceptable quality of life as they get older, and what seems unbearable to a 30-year-old seems fine to an 80-year-old, so that one has to be careful about decisions made too long in advance. But with the proviso that an advance directive would have to be updated or re-authenticated every three or five years or so, and with the proviso that there will always be circumstances which no form, however good, can possibly foresee, some kind of advance directive, ideally binding upon healthcare professionals, which makes it clear what an individual wants and does not want in extreme situations, would be very valuable.

It would, for instance, allow less intubation for those who find such treatment undignified. It would allow people to fade peacefully away with only pain relief. It would allow people to say they did not want to take the chemotherapy even though the chances of a beneficial outcome were relatively good, because at that stage of life the unpleasantness of the chemotherapy outweighed the value of a few more months of life. It would allow people to take charge of some of the circumstances of their own deaths, and that, whether one can tolerate the idea of euthanasia or not, must be of benefit.

Arguments against advance directives

There are those who would disapprove profoundly, who would say that each of us must have all possible life-saving treatments at all opportunities. In the

Jewish tradition, should it be that someone is dying and cannot be healed, the Jewish tradition comes unstuck. For we are not, on the whole, kind. We read, for instance, in a rabbinic collection (Ecclesiasticus Rabba v.6): 'Even when the physician realises that the end is nigh, he should order his patient to eat this and drink that, not eat this and not drink that. On no account should he tell him that the end is nigh'. We do not, traditionally, make the going easy. But one might reflect on why that should be. If human life is valued so highly, there is a clear reason to value every last moment of it, even if it is deeply uncomfortable, or one is in intense pain. That in itself throws an interesting sidelight on all the moves for assisted suicide, and euthanasia.

But, although one will find that attitude in many religious traditions, notably Judaism, Islam, and some forms of Christianity, nevertheless the majority of people are beginning to be seriously interested in advance directives or the appointment of a healthcare proxy. At the moment, no relative can make a decision for any other person, even if the person has appointed the brother or sister as a proxy. Technically, each of us has to give consent. Hence, apart from the desire to have advance directives which individuals fill in and discuss with their GPs, there is also a move to have the appointment of healthcare proxies who will have discussed these issues with their near and dear ones, and will know (as much as any other human being can know) what the person who is not competent to make a decision for themselves would have wanted. In the United States, this is now commonplace. In Britain, the move is only just beginning. But it has a value beyond that of advance directives, which are sensible in themselves.

The healthcare proxy

For the appointment of a healthcare proxy who will, *in extremis*, make healthcare decisions on one's behalf, including the decision to switch off life support, forces us all to talk to someone about these matters, something all too few of us do at present. If we are going to let someone else take these decisions on our behalf, we will have to discuss the issues of life and death – literally – with them. That discussion will have to include some of the more unpleasant aspects of what it can be like to die in certain circumstances, and what the person appointing the proxy actually wants to go through, and what not. For many of us, the thought remains that if we are dementing, with Alzheimer's disease or for whatever other reason, somehow there is no point going on living once we have anything remotely life-threatening anyway.

But it has to be said that there is a problem with this, which philosophers have been pointing out, which is that a person who is dementing with Alzheimer's can become, in a sense, a different person. Though it may seem infuriating to us if an elderly demented person says hello to the cat anew 600 times a day, that dementing older person may, in fact, have a new personality, may not be, in some sense, the same person as took the decision about an advance directive or healthcare proxy several years earlier. Thus, it may not be legitimate to take too seriously the views of someone who did not want anything to be done for them if they were dementing, when they have become a different person, staring out to sea from their porch, greeting the cat as an old friend repeatedly, apparently perfectly happy – but different.

This is the so-called incompetent patient, the one who is no longer able to make decisions for him- or herself. Someone has to take the decisions. The only debate is whether it should be the individual him- or herself in advance, if they get around to it, their nearest and dearest as a proxy, or the healthcare professionals acting in the 'best interests' of the patient, often with some sort of legal guardianship arrangement. Many of us will become 'incompetent'. Perhaps it is something that should be discussed in schools, so that children can become aware of the difficulties before they even have to begin to think about what it might be like for them, unless they are in the awful situation of a Tony Bland, or a young person with motor-cycle injuries, or whatever. But how we feel about our own 'incompetence', and how we wish to be treated, is still an open issue for debate.

These are not debates for healthcare professionals alone. These are debates, discussions, for all of us. But what we need to think about as we contemplate our end (even if it seems decades away) is what we really want, what we really believe is acceptable, whether we really believe our lives are our own, or are in God's hands, however we interpret that. Is this a matter for us as individuals? For society at large? For healthcare professionals? Should we be moving towards a more active euthanasia? Is it right to starve people? Should we be allowed to leave decision making, if we are incompetent, to our nearest and dearest? Can they genuinely be 'proxies' for us? Or have our perceptions changed?

There are probably no absolutely right answers here. Our technical capacities to keep people alive have outstripped our ability to think about these death issues clearly. So all we can do is the best we can, moving, as society has, towards regarding euthanasia, *in extremis,* as no bad thing.

7

The good death

All the previous chapters have argued that there are ways in which, in our society, we could approach death better. Most of the suggestions about how we might do it better have been essentially practical. It is not entirely a matter of attitude, though going into caring for dying people with the right attitude will help considerably. But it is also a matter of getting the practical details right. For instance, it is important to know enough about a dying person's culture or religion so as not to offend and so as to be able to offer something which might be of enormous significance – which one can only do with a little basic knowledge of the culture or religion from which the individual comes. Similarly, resolving some of the conflicts about decision making about how a person dies when the individual concerned can no longer make his or her wishes known easily, is another area where a little practical knowledge about asserting professional leadership can solve a lot of problems. So, too, can some knowledge of the psychology of grief help those who are bereaved come to terms with what they are feeling, and some minimal specialist knowledge about how children manifest grief differently from adults can also help parents of bereaved children cope.

These are not necessarily matters for intense deep thought – though individuals may choose to think long and hard about them. They are essentially areas where a little knowledge, which can be applied in given situations, might be very helpful. And the people who need that knowledge are not necessarily only healthcare professionals. The person who is dying might also wish to understand some of the practicalities. So, too, might the family concerned, as well as the clergy, the social workers, the teachers, indeed anyone in the community who might get involved with a family or an individual where there is a terminally ill person or a death has taken place. These are not matters for experts, but for all of us. Hence the simplicity of most of the messages this book contains, because they are messages for us all, not complicated, just practical.

For none of us is immune to the pain of death, so well prepared that the immediacy of shock and grief escape us. Even health professionals, supposedly able to be dispassionate about everything, can feel deeply moved and occasionally experience intense grief at the loss of a patient. I remember when I was a very junior rabbi going to see a member of my congregation who was in hospital. He had been very ill indeed, and had had a young nurse 'specialling' him, looking after him on a one-to-one basis. When I arrived, he had just died, and I found this young nurse in floods of tears in a linen cupboard. She had been told by her staff nurse that it was unprofessional for nurses to weep for their patients. I was shocked then, and I am still shocked recalling that incident. For a young nurse who has been looking after an elderly, very sick, very delightful man for some weeks is bound to get attached to him. Indeed, she would be a less good nurse if she did not, because some of her empathy would be missing. Why then, having spent so much time with him, should she not have felt bereft, sad at his loss, sad that they had not succeeded in enabling him to enjoy a few more years of life? Indeed, it was her very empathy, her affection for him, that had made him feel that he was being cherished in that huge ward. It was her very care which had made him feel it was worth at least trying to get better. She was right to feel upset. The staff nurse was wrong to be aggrieved at her behaviour – but the story tells us that there is still an attitude out there which suggests that health professionals should have no emotions, or, if they do, they should not show them.

Yet if health professionals are going to provide really top quality care, with empathy, they must have some emotional involvement with their patients. They cannot be immune. We should therefore be prepared to support them and to encourage them to express their emotions. Hence, not only should we provide the counselling as suggested in the previous chapter, but those of us who are not the professionals should also make a point of saying how sorry we are to the staff after they have been caring for someone who has died. We should empathise with the staff, as well as them empathising with the patient and the patient's family. Sometimes, it seems right for the family of someone who has died in a hospital or hospice to go back into the ward and chat to the staff who did the final caring, and talk through their shared grief. For the professionals and the family will have been involved together and, although the professionals will of necessity have moved on to caring for someone else, an important experience was nevertheless shared and it would be wrong to let it go without acknowledging the pain felt by family, friends and caring staff. Indeed, dealing with the pain can be very difficult. Grief takes one through many stages. But, somehow, each of those stages has to be marked by the family, the bereaved, and some of those stages may need to be marked by staff who were caring for the individual too. For instance, it is no bad thing if the member of healthcare staff who was 'specialling' a patient who was terminally ill actually attends the funeral. Not only will it often be comforting for the family to have the nurse or whoever there, but it may well also be helpful for the individual concerned to be present for the final public appearance, as it were, of the individual, to mark that stage of her or his own grief.

For grief is not an emotion to be ignored. It will not go away. It has to be worked through, be one widow or widower, family member, friend, carer, professional or otherwise. When grief is ignored, when for one reason or another someone who is upset, shocked, angry or pained by a death is forbidden to show it (as often used to happen with children and still occasionally does), then it will manifest itself later in different, abnormal ways. Instead of the stages of grief being gone through in the normal way, the anger, the upset, the misery, the depression, the final coming to terms, the anger will be contained and then may explode, or a clinical depression may ensue where it should not have done, or with children emotional development may cease or slow. The kinds of complications are varied and many, but the fact that grief is in any way not allowed to be expressed often means later difficulties.

Indeed, recognising the necessity of proper grieving and using such rituals as one's religion and culture provides, where they do, for staging the grief, leads to a resolution of grief. That is not to suggest that, at the end of the process, one suddenly feels it is all all right again, as if somehow the person who has died has come back to life. There is something macabre about the idea that 'it will all be all right soon', anyway. Yet, all too often that is what one hears said when well-meaning people are trying to bring comfort without knowing what to say. It will not be all right. It will be resolved, in some way, ending the agony of the pain. Most of us do learn to live again. But it is a different life with the loved one missing. Achieving a sense of it being worth-while to live again is what is essential. Finding a purpose, recognising a meaning, feeling a sense of sparkle, enjoying natural beauty, sensing the urgency of having to get back to work, are ways of feeling that life is worth living again. But it is not the same.

There is also, for many bereaved people, the sense that they have to carry on in order to look after children or aged parents. Young widows and widowers with children have to get on with living because of the children, yet they are all too often aware of how their children are grieving too – it is extremely difficult for them to support their children through their proper grief whilst they are grieving so intensely themselves, yet it is equally difficult for anyone but them to really talk to the children about the beloved parent. Equally, it is very difficult for someone elderly who is caring for a handi-capped child in middle age to express the intensity of his or her grief when often the middle-aged 'child' cannot quite grasp what is going on, and demands more attention even than usual. Nor is it easy for the extremely elderly widow or widower, whose family and friends often assume the pain of the grief will be less intense because the remaining spouse 'will be going to join' the one who has just died so soon. Sometimes, very elderly widowed people describe the comments of so-called comfort they get as a wish that they too would get on with the business of dying.

There are countless examples of where people, people like us, get the message wrong. The trick is not to make assumptions, but to listen. The Jewish tradition that one should visit the mourner but wait for the mourner to do the talking has some value to it, because by waiting for the mourner to speak one can get the right note in the music. But, in fact, many people stricken with grief find it hard to begin to speak at all, and we often have to begin for them, by asking them what we can do to help. Indeed, the offer of practical help, though all too often refused, is one way to begin a conversation with a bereaved person.

But the other important thing is to realise that often it does not much matter what we say. The important thing is that we are there, that we bother to say something at all. Even if all we say is that we are sorry for their troubles, or that we have heard about their loss and wish to express our sympathy, it is something. We have acknowledged their pain, their suffering, and their loss. We have made it clear we know that they will not be the same again. And we have registered that we will, in some way, be there for them. For bereaved people tell terrible tales of people crossing the street to avoid them because they do not know what to say. People who are dying, but still out and about in a wheelchair, for example, comment in the same way. People avoid them. With bereavement, the crossing of the road is surely done out of embarrassment, yet whatever the reason, it is unforgivable. The bereaved need the support of all of us who know them, and indeed even the support and recognition of those who do not really know them other than as acquaintances or neighbours. Grief needs recognition by a community, however private the emotion. Its very recognition (and hence widow's weeds and black-edged cards and the Jewish tradition of emptying containers of water) allows the bereaved people to behave differently, be supported, for a length of time. And that support, however difficult it is to give, allows the first stage of grieving to be done with recognition from one's fellow human beings that what one is experiencing is normal.

So grief can be used to draw people together within a community. Neighbours can club together to decorate the church for a funeral, to bring food for the family who are grieving, to take care of children and get them to school if they are going. More distant relatives and friends can even volunteer to stand with the children at the funeral, in case a widowed parent finds coping with the children's immediate reactions to the funeral too much to bear at the time. The grieving process can draw communities together, and more particularly families.

Yet it is no coincidence that the time of a death often drives families apart. People who rubbed along together perfectly happily for years suddenly find that the death of a key member brings out all the rivalries, all the factions, and not the love and fond memories. Wills, legacies, sharing out the spoils in the house, often make people behave incredibly badly. And those families who resolve never to fight about such things often deal with the difficulties by dividing things up in the oddest of ways. For instance, in my own family, my mother and her brother, who got on extremely well, decided to share their parents' possessions right down the middle. That meant splitting sets of cutlery, of glasses. Yet they continued that way, because they knew they absolutely did not wish to argue, and to say 'I would really like that set of knives...'. No – it is too unpleasant. Better funny half-sets of things than any kind of dispute. And that reaction is not unusual, because so many of us have seen the havoc a death, and spoils to be shared, has brought to an otherwise apparently harmonious wider family group.

Yet grief, bereavement and coping with the emotions after it, can and should be used to bring a family together. Clergy of all religions frequently have to deal with the complications of all this. They are often the ones who have to try to pour oil on troubled waters at the time of a death. They are also, as are hospice staff, the ones who have sometimes to try to sort out warring factions in families as they sit round the bedside of a dying person. Indeed, one hospice nurse told me an awful story of how she and one of the doctors and a member of the cleaning staff had to restrain two brothers who were coming to blows over the bed of their mother just as she was living her final few minutes!

That should not be necessary. Yet it is up to all of us, individuals involved, dying people ourselves with our families, clergy, social workers, health professionals and anyone else, to do our best to ensure that it does not happen. For the very strain of coping with terminal illness, the sheer exhaustion of caring for someone, and the nervous energy put into worrying, make the veneer of good behaviour wear very thin. Add to that the hope of inheritance, and the desire to have things belonging to the dear departed, and you have a recipe for family friction. It is therefore essential that we do everything in our power to prevent it.

There are various things we can do. First, the dying person can, him- or herself, make some fairly definitive statements about how he or she wants possessions shared out, to inhibit the fuss later. Secondly, the dying person can make it clear that he or she only wants to see a harmonious family at the side of the bed or wheelchair. Thirdly, they can say things to their children, assuming they are in their sixties or seventies or older, about the effect of the bickering on the grandchildren. Fourthly, they can encourage some straight talking between people who have had rows in the past – at the bedside. Those bedside reconciliations, the stuff of Victorian fiction, are in fact worth trying to engineer in some circumstances. Fifthly, the dying person can entrust a clergyperson, or a member of the caring team, to make clear certain wishes if he or she is no longer going to be able to do it. 'Your mother said I was to tell you...' is quite effective as a ruse to stop squabbling.

But these are practical suggestions to deal with the squabbling and rowing itself, unfortunately all too common. There are more complicated things we can try to do to change attitude, which relate more to how we view the death of a loved one than how to inhibit bad behaviour. For some people, the death of someone who has been ill is in itself a kind of resolution and often a relief. Sharing that relief, even though it has a sadness with it, even though there will be grieving to be done, is sometimes a way of bringing a family or community closer together. The sharing of genuine emotion, the talking about things that matter, either at the bedside or after a death, can bring families that have become distant from each other closer together. Indeed, if the families try hard to use the enforced space of the grieving process, the enforced time off work, the enforced time they have to spend together quietly, talking rather than sifting through papers or fighting about possessions, that time can itself be a time of healing, and can achieve precisely the kind of family bonding that is required to carry people thorough a hard time. But it requires a deliberate effort. And it requires one family member at least, if not more, to suggest that they use it for talking about important things, rather than hiding behind the fact (if it is a fact) that there is so much to do.

But that is the brave way to approach bringing the family and friends together after a death. It allows people to talk about the person who has died, which is very important to start the grieving process off. And it allows people to talk about things that matter to them in the family, even events that took place a long time ago. It can be enormously helpful, and it can strengthen family bonds, even though in most families there is a considerable amount of disapproval about what some members of the family have done at some stage.

But it is the effect of enforced time off work, enforced time to 'deal with' the business after someone has died, which allows resolution of feelings about each other. That is why a proper time for grieving is important, and it is why getting people together, waiting for people to come from abroad, is so important to the proper functioning of an extended family at the time of a death.

As the family is drawn together to mark the passing of someone, to go through at least part of the grieving process together, at least as far as the funeral is concerned and maybe a bit beyond, if there are mourning rituals beyond the funeral itself, such as a wake or evening prayers or a gathering at the gurdwara, they begin to give a shape to the grief itself. As a family unit, albeit an extended family, the shape of the grieving process and the shape of the family begin to enmesh. It is the people closest to the one who has died who feel the worst, but they are supported by the less close, who came for them, not for the one who has died, in many cases. The grieving rituals, if they are present, will be more intense for those who have the closest bonds with the one who had died, and it is the less close ones who will help the closer ones to do it. The shaping of grief is important, and the family support, and friends' support, is critical in allowing the grieving process to take its course, with gradually diminishing intensity.

But in order to do this effectively, some kind of grieving process needs to be in place. It need not be an ancient one. Many religions and cultures have ways of grieving, and these have been discussed in this book. But there are also plenty of modern groupings that have no ancient rituals, or have given them up. The Church of England is a good example of a religious organisation of some antiquity that has little in the way of grieving rituals beyond the funeral itself. In those circumstances, the family needs to sit down and think what it wants to do to give the grieving some shape, to think about whether there are ways of pacing the grief and things to do publicly to acknowledge one stage or another.

The classic example of that would be the memorial service. In many groupings, the memorial service is only a help for someone who had an important public life, who would have people who would want to pay their last respects to an individual (though in fact it is the family who appreciate it) and could not immediately be free to come to a funeral a few days after the death. So goes the thinking in many cases. There is also a tendency in modern Anglican families to have a family funeral only (and announcements saying family flowers only are increasingly frequent). If only family goes to the funeral, then there is often a large number of other people who want to mark the death in some way, for their own reasons, out of their own need to express their sorrow, to mark an end to a relationship. Thus, increasingly frequently, a memorial service is held some six or eight weeks after the death, announced in the newspaper, with a list of those who attended published shortly afterwards.

There is a confusion here. Family only funerals are all right in a way, but they exclude others who want to grieve. There are questions to be asked about the exclusivity of grief. Should immediate family exclude others who want to grieve from the funeral, on the basis that there will be a memorial service later? I am inclined to think that this may be unhealthy, and that the desire that others have to come and grieve should be respected.

It is different if the person was so public that thousands of admirers, hero-worshippers and journalists would want to be there. Then, there is an argument for keeping the grief to the family, and allowing those who are genuinely moved in a different way to have their private moment of mourning at the funeral. But those situations are rare. Most people, albeit relatively public figures, will not attract many strangers to their funerals. The people who are likely to want to come, but who may feel excluded, are those who worked with them, or those who loved them from a distance – friends, friends of the children or such like. There is something life-denying about families who exclude others from the funerals of their loved ones, as if to say that we, we only, loved this man or woman, and no-one who is not related can have a part in that. But in most cases, that is not true, and our relationships spread beyond our families into friendships with people of different worlds, and collegiality with people from work, relationships which were important during the deceased person's life, and which should not be denied now.

So there is an argument for allowing all who want to do so to come to a funeral. Yet often the funeral happens very quickly, in Jewish and Muslim families, in Irish families, Protestant or Catholic, often within 48 hours and sometimes within 24. In those circumstances, many who would have wanted to come will not even have heard about the death, as yet, and should, therefore, be given another opportunity. So memorial services have their place in allowing others a chance to express their grief.

They also do something else. When they are held for people who did not have an enormously important public life, though they made some kind of public contribution, six weeks or so after the death, they actually allow a different way of thinking about the person who has died to come to the fore. For the immediacy of the funeral still expresses the shock. In the funeral eulogy, although much will often be said about the person who has died, it will not be a memoir as such. At a memorial service it is possible to get a variety of different people who knew the person who died to talk about him or her from a personal perspective, and, when it is done well, you get a portrait of the person being drawn by different hands, and insights into their characters and lives that are intensely moving. It fulfils a different function then, one of remembering with affection as well as pain. For the first shock has gone, and the affectionate moments are being re-lived. It is a time when the grieving process has moved on, and can be very valuable for that reason alone, a good argument for encouraging memorial services where there is no wake or week of prayers, for example.

There is, too, an argument for those who have a religious faith to go to their place of worship regularly after the death has occurred. That is for several reasons. One is that it is probably part of the ritual anyway after a death. Another is that it gives the community a chance to support the bereaved, as most communities will wish to do. But the third reason is that, where there is no other obvious staging of grief, the use of weekly church attendance, say, or attendance at the gurdwara, allows the grief to be paced. There will be a gradual lessening of intensity. The nature of the pain, walking into the church with people staring and wondering what to say, will diminish, and the repetition of going weekly will allow the bereaved mourners to realise that there is a lessening of pain, albeit very gradual.

But much of this depends on realising that it is important to stage grief. Much of this depends on a public recognition that our grieving procedures leave much to be desired. We can look at traditional Jewish, Muslim, Irish, Hindu, and Sikh ways of coping with bereavement and know that there is something there which is worth emulating. But we cannot construct a grieving ritual out of nothing, nor can we explain the necessity for it, unless we talk more about death and its effects at times other than in the intensity of personal bereavement.

That is why I believe it is important that we talk about death with children in schools. It would be entirely possible, both in religious studies and in personal and social education, to make a study of how people talk about death and to encourage children to talk about their own experiences when, say, a grandparent died. It would of course have to be handled immensely sensitively. There may be children in a class who have lost a parent, or a grandparent. There may be children who have been bereaved and whose own need to grieve was not recognised. There is all too likely to be a child in the class whose parents did not know how to mark the stages of grief, because that is a common English phenomenon (much less common in Scotland, Wales and Ireland, north and south). Those difficulties will need to be handled. There is no point in a teacher jumping into a minefield like this with two left feet. Children will have to be asked gently about their experiences. They will have to be encouraged to think of times of death in literature, or on TV. They will need to try to make personal references to what they have heard about people dying, and people being bereaved. But having it on the syllabus, having it within the curriculum, will at least allow the sort of discussion we should all have had as teenagers or slightly older, about what we feel about death ourselves, and how best we can encourage others to grieve well, and learn to grieve well ourselves.

There are strong moves to have education about parenting for children in schools, partly because the experience of child abuse suggests that abused children often become abusers themselves. If there are strong moves to have education about parenting in our schools, then there is as much need to have education about death and dying in our schools, to enable people to think about the effects of a death, and about ways of marking the death of someone they love. For the evidence of damage to children who are not allowed to grieve is considerable, and it cannot be beyond the capacities of our education system to encourage children to think about death and dying, and to work out how they would like to be allowed to grieve. For it will only be as a result of encouraging the next generation to think about grieving that we might, gradually, introduce back into English practice, around the time of a death, a ritualising of the grieving process which allows the pacing to take place.

That is one very good reason for teaching children, and encouraging children to discuss the ways people mourn. But there are other reasons, one at least of which is to discourage a fear of death in them. Many children, many schools, help in local hospices. Children are much more likely now than 10 years ago to go into a hospice and see people who are dying, one thing in itself which will discourage their fear. But beyond that, they could discuss the hospice idea in the classroom, and they could think about what it means to simply cease to exist, as well as discussing, in religious studies at least, different religions' ideas about what happens after death. Since we know that children worry about death, since we know that young bereaved people suffer considerably, there really is a strong argument for discussing death and dying in the course of general education for all children. It could be both challenging and comforting, and it might be therapeutic if, as a result of discussion, young people felt that we could learn to die better, and grieve better, in Britain.

Part of that could be achieved by acquiring a better language of grief. We use grief, and talk of stages of grief, because we cannot differentiate all that easily between the various stages except by quite lengthy explanations. We have no equivalent of the different terms used for the various stages of grief by other religions and cultures. My own religion has the shiva, the seven days, followed by the shloshim, the 30 days, followed by 11 months. Sikhism has the 10 days marked by a ceremony and a reading of the Guru Granth Sahib. Irish Catholicism has the removal of the body, the funeral mass, and the burial, and the saying of masses in memory of the dead. Yet the usual thing is to find in most cultures and religions that there is much less differen-tiation of the stages. It is therefore essential that, as we find it easier to talk about these things, as, in the new millennium, death stops being the great unmentionable that it was for much of the latter part of the 20th century, that we develop a vocabulary to talk about grief and loss.

Some of that has come about through the work of the psychologists who have concentrated their efforts on looking at loss and grief. But far more needs to be done on a much wider stage than has been achieved thus far. People need to be able to say, to their intimates at least, I am in the gut-wrenching stages of grief, to the extent that I have physical pain – but using different terms. They need to be able to talk about the calm after the storm of weeping, until another wave hits. They need to be able to talk about the anger most bereaved people feel, which has a different quality to it from that of other forms of anger, and needs to be described differently, if at all possible. So it is not easy to work out how to establish a new language of grief, but it is vital, so that all of us can talk more easily about how we feel, and so that bereavement counsellors, who now talk, and listen, so much to those who are bereaved, can talk with people who are better informed about the feelings they are going through, and what is normal and what is not.

If we can achieve this, if we can ensure that most ordinary people know something about how we grieve, what happens, what is normal, what is not, so that bereavement can be seen as something most of us go through at some stage in our lives, as normal as falling in love, or having children, part of life's progress, then we will begin to have a much more natural, less denying, approach to the whole business of death and dying. For if we can take bereavement as a normal state for most of us, at some stage in our lives, one of the prices we pay for loving, then we can begin to think in a more natural way about the implications of dying, and think more, too, about how we wish to face our own ends, should we have any control over the matter.

That means thinking more about the idea of the good death. Do we want to die with our family all round us? Do we want to have an official final conver-sation with each member of our family? Do we want to make a final trip to a beloved place, or to see a beloved painting, or hear beloved music? Do we want to stay at home and die in our own surroundings, cared for by those we love and who love us, or is that too much of a burden to place upon them? Do we want to die in a hospice where the knowledge about pain control, quite apart from the knowledge about emotional reactions to death, is so very great, so that we will experience no pain? Do we want to die by jumping under a train? (It has always seemed to me that such a way of committing suicide is unfair to the driver, who has no reason to be drawn into one's private agony.) Is there a point at which we want to tolerate no more?

These are important questions. We vary considerably in how we feel about them. Yet, if we wish to establish the good death, at a time when it is quite easy to keep many of us alive, in some shape or form, for far longer than it was in the 18th century (when we would have lain in bed and had laudanum to rid us of the pain, and shortened our lives as a result, with no-one thinking any the worse of us for doing it), we have to think about it. We have to ask ourselves these questions. We have to discuss them with our nearest and dearest. We have to make sure that our spouses and/or children know what we feel.

But we need to wrestle with our consciences. Are we going to take the purist line Judaism and Islam would take, that one must do absolutely nothing to shorten life in any way, even if the rest of one's life is painful and distressing, because life is God's gift? Or are we going to say that anything we can do to rid ourselves of pain and to allow ourselves to die in dignity, short of actually committing suicide, is permissible?

There are no clear answers to these questions. Each of us will answer them in different ways. We will all have to examine our consciences whilst we think about how important every last minute of life is to us. But we will also have to think about the implications of the good death, dying well being one way we will be remembered by those who come after us, dying with dignity, able to say our goodbyes without needing to be watched as we disappear into a huddle of shrieking senility or intractable pain. It is a personal matter, but one that we cannot leave until the time. It is a personal matter to be thought about in youth and then again all one's life until one comes to the time when the question becomes a reality.

We can see some people die with great dignity. I have never forgotten a young Buddhist man in considerable pain, who died not wanting to take opiate pain-killing drugs because of the way they would cloud his vision. He was determined to reach the highest stage of consciousness as he approached his death, knowing he was to die in the next few days. He must have been in agony, but, apart from the strained expression around his eyes, you would not have been able to tell. He struggled with his awareness, because he was sure that the right way to die was to meet one's maker in a heightened stage of awareness, on a spiritual high, so to speak. He discussed this with his family and friends, the friends from the commune he was living in. They brought him a Buddhist monk to discuss things with, and he talked to him for a relatively short time. The various friends came and read a variety of holy books to him, and he seemed to relax, and would then ask a question about the meaning of something he had heard.

Or, there was the young woman, a committed Anglican, who was dying of bony metastases after a peculiarly horrible and virulent primary breast cancer. She discussed her feelings with her clergyman. She asked to see a deaconess (this was before there were women priests in the Church of England), because she wanted to talk about the particularly female nature of the disease. She took plenty of pain-relieving drugs, which worked less than well. Yet she wanted to pray, to hear Psalms read, to meet her maker in resignation and with acceptance.

Those were, for those people, good deaths, death met as they had wished it to be. It is in contrast with the people who fight all the way, not accepting their fate. I remember a middle-aged man dying of cancer, a Jew, who refused to believe it. He had too much to do in his life, he was nowhere near the end of his agenda, it was not fair, it was unreasonable. 'Try anything, doctor. Is there nothing new, nothing experimental you can give me...?' He refused to believe it, and would not go quietly. Yet, his doctors said afterwards, his very reluctance to go had probably allowed him to stay alive, and have a reasonable quality of life, for all but his last few weeks anyway. Yet that could hardly be called a good death, except insofar as it allowed him to have what he wanted, which was as much time as was remotely possible.

People vary dramatically in how they choose to have the good death. Some see themselves as having the good death if they are literally surrounded by their family as they make their goodbyes, rather like those pictures of deathbed scenes in late 18th and early 19th century studies. Whatever the pattern, however much it complies with older versions of the good death, or is a newer version in accordance with the individual's wishes, it is likely to be a better death if he or she has discussed it with the rest of their family, or a spouse or child at least, so that as much as possible can be in accordance with his or her wishes. It also allows for it to be a death which is, to some extent at least, at peace, in reconciliation, where everyone around is aware that this was the way the dying person wanted to go, and has done as much as they could to make that possible. The good death may be nothing like 18th century ideals, but if it is one which has been discussed, even planned for, with as much as possible achieved as could be, given the constraints, that might then be the modern equivalent of the good death.

For now we have a host of disciplines to play with, which our 18th century ancestors did not have at their disposal. They had religion, although the 18th century was the first really questioning age. But they did not have psychology, where a study of human reactions can be so very useful. Their medical skills were also nowhere near as good as ours, although, sometimes, we may challenge what is done in the name of medicine, of science, at the end of life. Nor were they very interested in questions of diversity of culture. The society was much more culturally uniform, and now we have things to learn from the various communities in our midst, things which can be extremely enriching when we examine how other peoples, other religious groupings, people whose origins may have been, say, in the Indian sub-continent, think differently about death and about bereavement. We can learn from the communities amongst whom we live, and we can add to our own traditions, and to other people's, by thinking hard how we would most like to die and how we would grieve most healthily, with the least lasting damage psychologically speaking.

If we can learn from all our newer disciplines, from the cultures in our midst and elsewhere in the world, and from some understanding of spirituality within or outside the framework of organised religion, we may be able to die better ourselves, if we face the inevitable questions. Whether we do better for ourselves or not, however, by thinking about these issues, and by learning from the various disciplines around us, which have useful things to contribute, we can certainly provide a better death for those for whom we are caring, whether they are members of our families, our friends, our patients or our clients. We can bring better understanding to the task, and we can ensure that the people who are dying get as much out of the experience as possible, that the very act of dying seems to them, and to us, in some way life-enhancing. For, that way, we can see a real cycle of growth and decay, of life and death, and we can watch people die and know that others will look after us as gently and supportively as we looked after those people, and that their children will look after our children, and so on. But we will only die better, and grieve better, if we are now prepared to talk about it beyond the confines of the hospice movement, in our homes, our schools, our churches, mosques, gurdwara, temples and synagogues. We will only achieve a real change, allowing ourselves to express our fears and hopes and desires, if we are prepared to face the issue of how best to meet our end and to face the end of others we love and respect, by discussing, by talking, by arguing, by planning, and by resolving to improve what is still a very patchy situation in the UK, particularly if we are dying of anything other than cancer.

Some years ago, caring for dying people was something people did not talk about. The hospice movement has transformed that attitude. But it has not yet normalised the dying process for us all, nor really given thought to how the dying person can drive the way he or she wants to be cared for, if they do not wholly share the hospice philosophy. Freedom from pain is what most dying people want. Many want to die at home, if at all possible. But not everyone wants the calm of mind, the spiritual care, that a hospice provides. And we need to take note of the very different requirements of many different people in our society, and let them tell us how they would most like to be cared for. And, for that, we need a public debate that goes beyond euthanasia, advance directives and healthcare proxies. We need a recognition of the pain of separation, the pain of loss, the pain of finality, and we need to bring death and dying into everyday discussions – at school, at universities and, of course, in the media.

Only then will we begin to wrestle towards a good death for everyone, whatever we are dying from, however old we are, however we want it, helped, but not limited, by the professionals. Only then will we have a sense that the Good Death Guide will not be long in coming, modelled on the Good Birth Guide. For our dying should be the last human endeavour over which we can have control – doing it our way.

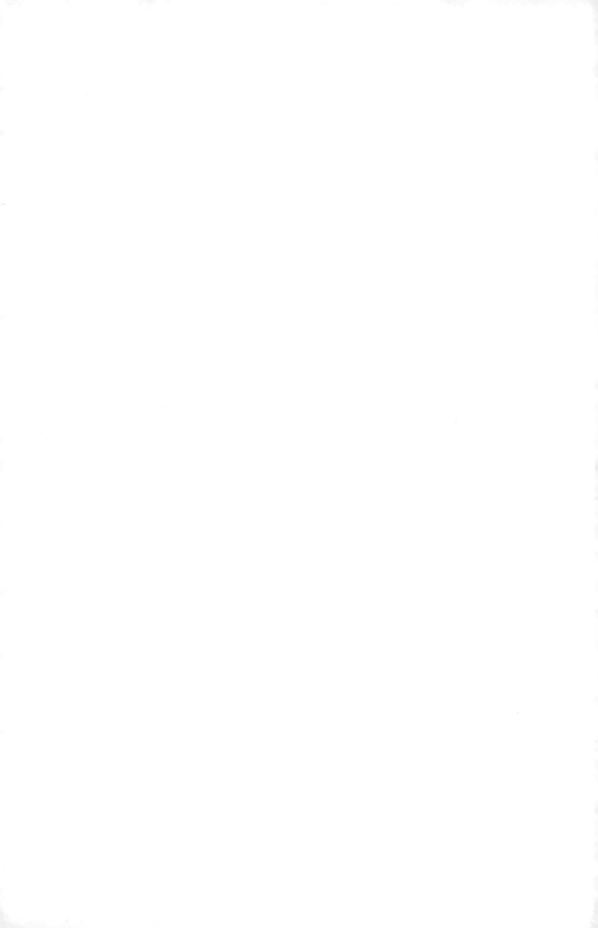

General information and bibliography

Useful addresses

Hospital Chaplaincies Council
Church House
Great Smith Street
London SW1P 3NZ
Tel: 020 7898 1894
Fax: 020 7898 1891

National Council for Hospice and Specialist Palliative Care Services
34–44 Britannia Street
London WC1X 9JG
Tel: 020 7520 8299

Hospice Information Service
St Christopher's Hospice
51–59 Lawrie Park Road
London SE26 6DZ
Tel: 020 8778 9252

Cruse Bereavement Care
Cruse House
126 Sheen Road
Richmond
Surrey TW9 1UR

Tel: 020 8940 4818
Helpline: 020 8332 7227

The Buddhist Hospice Trust
Website: www.buddhisthospice.org.uk

CancerBACUP
3 Bath Place
Rivington Street
London EC2A 3DR
Tel: 020 7696 9003
Helpline: 0808 800 1234
Email: info@cancerbacup.org.uk

Child Death Helpline
Bereavement Services Department
Great Ormond Street Hospital NHS Trust
Great Ormond Street
London WC1N 3JH
Tel: 020 7813 8551
Helpline: 0800 282 986

The Compassionate Friends
53 North Street
Bristol BS3 1EN
Tel: 0117 966 5202
Helpline: 0117 953 9639

Macmillan Cancer Relief
89 Albert Embankment
London SE1 7UQ
Tel: 020 7840 7840
Information line: 0845 601 6161
Website: www.macmillan.org.uk

The Natural Death Centre
6 Blackstock Mews
Blackstock Road
London N4 2BT
Tel: 020 7359 8391
Email: rhino@dial.pipex.com
Website: www.naturaldeath.org.uk

Useful reading

If you read nothing else, read Michael Waterhouse's *Staying Close: a positive approach to dying and bereavement* (Constable 2003). It summarises the classic texts beautifully, and it contains much useful material by someone who wrote the book after his mother's death of motor neurone disease, having long been a television producer, particularly of religious programmes.

My own work *Caring for Dying People of Different Faiths* (Radcliffe Medical Press 2004) may also be useful, and I would never be without a copy of the *Encyclopedia of Death and Dying*, edited by Glennys Howarth and Oliver Leaman ((Routledge 2001).

A full bibliography follows.

Bibliography

Ainsworth-Smith I and Speck P (1982) *Letting Go: caring for the dying and bereaved*. SPCK, London.

Argyle M and Beit-Hallahmi B (1975) *The Social Psychology of Religion*. Routledge and Kegan-Paul, London.

Barker P (1996) *The Ghost Road*. Penguin, Harmondsworth.

Beauchamp TL and Childress JF (1989) *Principles of Biomedical Ethics* (3e). Oxford University Press, Oxford and New York.

Black D (1999) *When Patients Die: learning to live with the loss of a patient*. Routledge, London.

Boston S and Tresize R (1987) *Merely Mortal: coping with dying, death and bereavement*. Channel Four, Methuen, London.

Bowlby J (1974) *Attachment and Loss*. Hogarth, London.

Brittain V (1978) *Testament of Youth*. Virago Press, London.

Brontë C (1994) *Jane Eyre*. Penguin, Harmondsworth.

Burkhardt VR (1982) Chinese Creeds and Customs. *South China Morning Post*, Hong Kong.

Burleigh M (1994) *Death and Deliverance – Euthanasia in Germany 1900–1945*. Cambridge University Press, Cambridge.

Campbell A (1981) *Rediscovering Pastoral Care*. Darton, Longman and Todd, London.

Carroll P (2002) Euthanasia: reflecting on the experience of dying. *Journal of Community Nursing*. **16**(11): 37–9.

Clements E (2000) Society and Death. *Journal of Community Nursing*. Dec **14**(12): 6–10.

Cobb M and Robshaw V (eds) (1998) *The Spiritual Challenge of Health Care*. Churchill Livingstone, Edinburgh.

Cobb M (2001) Walking on Water? The moral foundations of chaplaincy. In: H Orchard (ed.) *Spirituality in Health Care Contexts* Jessica Kingsley, London.

Crichton I (1976) *The Art of Dying*. Brill Academic Publisher, Leiden.

Dein S and George R (2001) The time to die: symbolic factors relating to the time of death. *Mortality*. **6**(2): 203–11.

Dinnage R (1990) *The Ruffian on the Stair*. Viking, London.

Downie RS and Calman KC (1987) Healthy Respect – ethics in healthcare. Oxford University Press, London.

Enright DJ (1983) *The Oxford Book of Death*. Oxford University Press, Oxford.

Firth S (2001) *Wider Horizons: care of the dying in a multicultural society*. National Council for Hospice and Specialist Palliative Care Services, London.

Freud S (1917) Mourning and Melancholia. In: S Freud (1953) *Collected Papers* (Vol. 4). Hogarth, London.

Van Gennep A (1960) *Rites of Passage*. University of Chicago Press, Chicago and Routledge, London.

Goffman E (1990) *Stigma: notes on the management of spoiled identity*. Penguin, Harmondsworth.

Goffman E (1985) *Behaviour in Public Places*. The Free Press, London.

Gorer G (1965) *Death, Grief and Mourning in Contemporary Britain*. Cresset Press, London.

Gorovitz S (1991) *Drawing the Line: life, death and ethical choices in an American hospital*. Oxford University Press, New York and Oxford.

Graham J, Ramirez AJ, Cull A *et al.* (1996) Job stress and satisfaction among palliative physicians. *Pall Med*. **10**: 185–94.

Grof S and Halifax J (1978) *The Human Encounter with Death*. Souvenir Press, London.

Hart B, Sainsbury P and Short S (1998) Whose Dying? A sociological critique of the 'good death'. *Mortality*. **3**(1): 65–77.

Henley A (1982–84) *Asians in Britain* (3 vols). *Caring for Sikhs and their Families: religious aspects of care. Caring for Muslims and their Families: religious aspects of care. Caring for Hindus and their Families: religious aspects of care*. DHSS and King Edward's Hospital Fund for London, National Extension College, London.

Hinton J (1967) *Dying*. Penguin, Harmondsworth.

Howarth G and Leaman O (eds) (2001) *Encyclopedia of Death and Dying*. Routledge, London.

Iqbal M (1981) *East Meets West* (3e). Commission for Racial Equality, London.

Klein M (1940) Mourning and its relation to manic depressive states. *Int J Psycho Anal*. **21**: 125–53.

Klein M (1975) Our adult world and its roots in infancy. In: *Envy and Gratitude*. Karnac Books, London.

Klein M (1937) Love, Hate and Reparation. Hogarth, London.

Kubler-Ross E (1970) *On Death and Dying*. Tavistock, London.

Kung H and Jens W (1995) A Dignified Dying: a plea for personal responsibility. SCM Press, London.

Lamm M (1969) *The Jewish Way in Death and Mourning*. Jonathan David, New York.

Lewis CS (1961) *A Grief Observed*. Faber, London.

Lindemann E (1944) The symptomatology and management of acute grief. *Am J Psych*. **September**: 7f.

Locke DC (1992) *Increasing Multicultural Understanding – a comprehensive model*. Sage Publications, Newbury Park, Calif.

Lothian Community Relations Council (1984) *Religions and Cultures: a guide to patients' beliefs and customs for health service staff*. Lothian Community Relations Council, Edinburgh.

Masson JD (2002) Non-professional perceptions of 'good death': a study of the views of hospice care patients and relatives of deceased hospice care patients. *Mortality*. **7**(2): 191–209.

McGilloway O and Myco F (eds) (1985) *Nursing and Spiritual Care*. Harper and Row, London.

Mitford J (1978) *The American Way of Death*. Simon and Schuster, New York.

Moberg DO (1973) Religiosity in old age. In: L Brown (ed.) *Psychology and Religion*. Penguin, Harmondsworth.

Moggach D (1994) And Now I Miss the Rest of Me. *The Times*, 19 February.

Neuberger J (1994) *Caring for Dying Patients of Different Faiths*. Mosby, London.

Neuberger J and White J (eds) (1991) *A Necessary End*. Macmillan, London.

Noll P (1989) *In the Face of Death*. Viking, Harmondsworth.

Nuland S (1994) *How We Die*. Chatto & Windus, London.

Orchard H (ed.) (2001) *Spirituality in Health Care Contexts*. Jessica Kingsley, London.

Parkes CM (1972) *Bereavement*. Penguin, Harmondsworth.

Payne SA, Langley-Evans A and Hillier R (1996) Perceptions of a 'good' death: a comparative study of the views of hospice staff and patients. *Pall Med*. **10**: 307–12.

Pincus L (1976) *Death and the Family*. Faber, London.

Porter R and Porter D (1988) *In Sickness and in Health, the British Experience 1650–1850*. Fourth Estate, London.

Rees D (1997) *Death and Bereavement: the psychological, religious and cultural interfaces*. Whurr publishers, London.

Riemer J (eds) (1974) *Jewish Reflections on Death*. Schocken Books, New York.

Rosenblatt PC (2002) Grief in families. *Mortality*. **7**(2): 125–7.

Royal College of Physicians (1990) *Research Involving Patients*. Royal College of Physicians, London.

Sampson C (1982) *The Neglected Ethic: religious and cultural factors in the care of patients*. McGraw-Hill, Maidenhead.

Saunders C, Summers DH and Teller N (1981) *Hospice: the living idea*. Edward Arnold, London.

Spiegel Y (1977) *The Grief Process: analysis and counselling*. SCM Press, London.

Taylor T (2002) *The Buried Soul: how humans invented death*. Fourth Estate, London.

Thielicke H (1983) *Living with Death*. Eerdmans, Grand Rapids.

Vincent S (1994) Exits. *Guardian Weekend*, 19 February.

Walter T (1994) *The Revival of Death*. Routledge, London.

Waterhouse M (2003) *Staying Close: a positive approach to dying and bereavement*. Constable, London.

Winterson J (1991) *Oranges are not the Only Fruit*. Vintage, London

Young M and Cullen L (1996) *A Good Death: conversations with East Londoners*. Routledge, London.

Index